Growing Older

Growing older in Europe

Growing Older

Series Editor: Alan Walker

The objective of this series is to showcase the major outputs from the ESRC Growing Older programme and to provide research insights that will result in improved policy and practice and enhanced and extended quality of life for older people.

It is well known that people are living longer but until now very little attention has been given to the factors that determine the quality of life experienced by older people. This important new series will be vital reading for a broad audience of policy makers, social gerontologists, nurses, social workers, sociologists and social geographers as well as advanced undergraduate and postgraduate students in these disciplines.

Series titles include:

Ann Bowling *Ageing Well*

Joanne Cook, Tony Maltby and Lorna Warren *Older Women's Lives*

Maria Evandrou and Karen Glaser *Family, Work and Quality of Life for Older People*

Mary Maynard, Haleh Afshar, Myfanwy Franks and Sharon Wray *Women in Later Life*

Sheila Peace, Caroline Holland and Leonie Kellaher *Environment and Identity in Later Life*

Thomas Scharf, Chris Phillipson and Allison E Smith *Ageing in the City*

Christina Victor, Sasha Scambler and John Bond *The Social World of Older People*

Alan Walker (ed.) *Growing Older in Europe*

Alan Walker and Catherine Hagan Hennessy (eds) *Growing Older: Quality of Life in Old Age*

Alan Walker (ed.) *Understanding Quality of Life in Old Age*

Growing Older

Growing older in Europe

edited by
Alan Walker

Open University Press

Open University Press
McGraw-Hill Education
McGraw-Hill House
Shoppenhangers Road
Maidenhead
Berkshire
England
SL6 2QL
email: enquiries@openup.co.uk
world wide web: www.openup.co.uk

and Two Penn Plaza, New York, NY 10121–2289, USA

First published 2005
Copyright © Alan Walker 2005

A catalogue record of this book is available from the British Library

ISBN 0335 21513 0 (pb) 0335 21514 9 (hb)

Library of Congress Cataloguing-in-Publication data
CIP data applied for

Typeset by RefineCatch Ltd, Bungay, Suffolk
Printed in the UK by MPG Books, Bodmin

Contents

Contributors

Lars Andersson, Institute for the Study of Ageing and Later Life (ISAL), Linköping University, Norrköping, Sweden
http://www.ituf.liu.se/tema_ae/startpage

Beitske Bouwman, Department of Social Cultural Studies, section Social Gerontology, Free University, Amsterdam, The Netherlands

Kees Knipscheer, Department of Social Cultural Studies, section Social Gerontology, Free University, Amsterdam, The Netherlands
http://www.ssg.scw.vw.nl/lasa

Giovanni Lamura, INRCA, Department of Gerontological Research, Ancona, Italy
http://www.inrca.it/CES/CVenglish.pdf

Annemarie Peeters, Department of Social Cultural Studies, section Social Gerontology, Free University, Amsterdam, The Netherlands

Francesca Polverini, INRCA, Department of Gerontological Research, Ancona, Italy

Monika Reichert, Institute of Sociology, University of Dortmund, Dortmund, Germany
http://www.fb12.uni-dortmund.de/stat/soziologie/Soziologie.htm

Alan Walker, Department of Sociological Studies, University of Sheffield,
http://www.shef.ac.uk/socst/staff/a_walker.htm
http://www.shef.ac.uk/uni/projects/gop/

Carol Walker, Department of Policy Studies, University of Lincoln

Manuela Weidekamp-Maicher, Institute for Gerontology at the University of Dortmund, Dortmund, Germany
http://www.uni-dortmund.de/FFG

Preface

The origins of this book lie in the specification for the Economic and Social Research Council's (ESRC) Growing Older (GO) programme. When, in 1997, I was asked to prepare a proposal for a programme of research on extending quality of life to go to the ESRC's Research Priorities Board, I argued that the programme should contain a major European comparative dimension. When the GO programme was approved and funded by the ESRC the European component was deleted for cost reasons. Subsequently I applied for funding under the EU's Fifth Framework programme, Key Action 6 on the Ageing Population and Disabilities, for a small Accompanying Measure project to create the European dimension of the GO programme. This project commenced in October 2001 and culminated in a workshop on Quality of Life in Old Age, in London, in June 2002. It consisted of five national research reviews on the current knowledge about quality of life in old age in Germany, Italy, the Netherlands, Sweden and the UK. This work, revised and updated, comprises the bulk of this book, together with an introductory overview. It is published in the GO series as the European companion to the two edited volumes that report the key findings from the programme.

Thanks go to the ESRC for funding the GO programme and, specifically, to Faye Auty for her help as the first programme officer; to the European Commission for funding the EQUAL-AGE Accompanying Measure (QLK6–CT–2001–30168), particularly to Peter Kind for his encouragement and support; and to Georgios Mezelas, Gabriel Karajian, Hans-Juergen Jaeckel, Analisa Colosimo and Maria Theofilatou for their administrative backup. Thanks to the participants in the London workshop who helped to sharpen some of the arguments contained in this book and, especially to Rocio Fernandez Ballesteros and Ann Bowling for their comments on a draft of Chapter 1. At the University of Sheffield, thanks to Gill Wells for her help with the EQUAL contract and finances, to Catherine Hennessy and Jo Levesley for help with the workshop and its report, to Marg Walker for her invaluable support to both the GO programme and the EQUAL-AGE Project and for preparing this book for publication, and to Alison Ball for her work on the book. Special thanks go to Carol Walker for her help and support. Finally the book is dedicated to Anne-Marie Guillemard for her scientific inspiration and for introducing me to comparative European research on ageing.

Alan Walker
University of Sheffield

To Anne-Marie Guillemard

1

Quality of life in old age in Europe

Alan Walker

Introduction

This chapter provides an overview of the research reported in the rest of the book, which is based on systematic reviews of the current state of knowledge regarding quality of life (QoL) in old age in the five European Union (EU) countries represented here. Its main aim is to highlight the key factors identified by the national experts as determining QoL.

All of the work contained in this book derives from the EU funded EQUAL project. This was an 'Accompanying Measure' under the Fifth Framework programme. A central focus of Key Action 6 of the programme – the ageing population and disabilities – was on reducing morbidity and coping with disability to extend quality life in old age and enhance the functional independence of older people. A wide range of new research was commissioned to reflect the objectives of the Key Action. However, this small project was based on existing research with the specific intention of surveying the current state of knowledge in order, first, to assess what is known about QoL in old age, second, to disseminate information between member states and, third, to identify gaps in research on this topic.

The range of European countries represented was heavily constrained by the budget available and the five chosen were intended to represent a variety of EU national and institutional contexts: north/south, large/small, centralized/ decentralized and, in terms of welfare states, Beveridge, Bismarck and hybrid types. The countries covered are Germany, Italy, the Netherlands, Sweden and the UK (with the UK contribution being purposely summary in relation to the others, because of the ready availability of information on the UK in other

books in this series, and heavily reliant on the Growing Older [GO] programme). The contributors were asked to review the existing knowledge in
their countries on the factors that extend or limit QoL among older people.
Drafts of these reviews were discussed extensively at a workshop, in London, in
June 2002. The revised and updated versions are contained in this book with
two chapters representing each country.

To encourage standardization and to facilitate comparisons between countries each chapter follows a common pattern. Part I of the book focuses on
definitional issues, environmental and socio-economic aspects of QoL in old
age. Each chapter covers four key topics:

- definition and measurement of QoL;
- environment, housing, neighbourhood, transport, new technology;
- physical and mental health;
- employment and income.

Part II deals primarily with the relational and participative aspects of the
quality of later life and each chapter covers five key topics:

- family and support networks;
- participation and social integration;
- role of services in QoL;
- life satisfaction and subjective wellbeing;
- inequalities/variations in QoL.

In addition the contributors were asked to identify significant gaps in research.
The EQUAL project formed the European partner to the UK GO programme, which was funded by the ESRC and was aimed at generating
new knowledge about the factors that determine quality in later life
(http://www.shef.ac.uk/uni/projects/gop/index.htm). Thus this book should
be read in conjunction particularly with the two edited volumes that report
the findings of the GO Programme and which represent the state-of-the-art
research on QoL in old age in the UK (Walker and Hagan Hennessy 2004;
Walker, 2005).

Ageing Europe

A brief overview of demographic structure and change in Europe will provide
a context for the comparative synthesis of the analyses of QoL in the five EU

countries represented in this book. Most of the statistics that follow refer to the 15 EU member states up to May 2004 and exclude the ten new ones that joined on 1 May. It is well known that the EU is ageing and, indeed, is already the world's oldest region (Walker and Maltby 1997). In 2000 there were 61 million people aged 65 and over in the EU – 16 per cent of the total population – compared with 34 million in 1960 (European Commission 2003).

There are two key drivers of population ageing: the decline in fertility rates to below replacement levels and a fall in mortality. In addition there is a historically unique event impending with the approach to retirement of the cohort born immediately after the Second World War – the baby boomers. Fertility has been dropping in the EU for four decades but, remarkably, 2000 recorded the highest number of births for six years. The total fertility rate for the EU increased from 1.45 children per woman in 1999 to 1.53 in 2000 but still remains low in historical terms. Only in Germany and the UK did the rate continue to decrease in 2000. The lowest fertility levels are in Italy and Spain and the social importance of this demographic fact, in a southern European country particularly when coupled with south to north migration, is discussed in Chapters 3 and 8. As far as the ten new member states are concerned only Cyprus (1.83) currently exceeds the average fertility rate for the EU-15 (1.53), while the Czech Republic has the lowest rate of all countries (1.14).

At the same time as fertility has declined, life expectancy has increased by about ten years over the last 50 years, a phenomenon that is even more remarkable because of the linear nature of the average increase, which stretches back to the 1840s (Oeuppen and Vaupel 2002). Table 1.1 shows that average life expectancy for women in the EU-15 exceeds 80 years while men continue to lag behind by more than six years on average.

In the four decades since the 1960s the proportion of people aged 65 and over has risen from 11 per cent to 16 per cent of the EU total population. A continuation of this trend is expected and, between 2005 and 2020, the population aged 65 and over will increase by 22 per cent. Growth will be over 30 per cent in Ireland, Luxembourg, the Netherlands and Finland and will be below 20 per cent in Belgium, Spain, Portugal and the UK. Women will continue to outnumber men, by a ratio of roughly three to two.

As Table 1.2 shows the very elderly or 'old-old', those aged 80 and over, currently comprise nearly 4 per cent of the total population of the EU-15. Over the next 15 years the numbers in this age group will rise by almost 50 per cent (European Commission 2003). The rate of increase varies considerably across the EU reaching as much as 70 per cent in Greece but is below 10 per cent in

3

Table 1.1 Life expectancy at birth, 1999

	Men	Women
Austria	74.4	80.9
Belgium	74.3	80.5
Denmark	74.0	78.8
Finland	73.7	81.0
France	74.9	82.3
Germany	74.5	80.6
Greece	75.5	80.6
Ireland	73.5	79.1
Italy	75.5	81.8
Luxembourg	73.7	80.5
Netherlands	75.2	80.5
Portugal	71.7	78.9
Spain	75.3	82.5
Sweden	77.1	81.9
UK	74.8	79.7
EU-15	74.6	80.9

Source: European Commission (2003)

Denmark and Sweden. Those over the age of 80 are predominantly women, by a ratio of more than two to one, and they are most prone to disability and to higher than average use of health and social services, and are most likely to be living alone – key issues that are explored in detail in the subsequent chapters. Table 1.2 also shows that the ten new EU member states are 'younger' than the existing ones in having lower proportions in the very elderly age group. Three of the five countries under consideration in this book have above average percentages aged 80 and over, the two exceptions being Germany and the Netherlands. Sweden and the UK lead the EU in this respect.

National data conceal fact that population ageing is a local and regional issue. In some parts of Europe, where ageing is coupled with the out migration of younger age groups, older people will soon be the majority – for example in parts of southern Italy, central France and northern Spain. The variations

Table 1.2 Population structure, 2000

	0 – 19	20 – 59	60 – 79	80 and over	Total
Austria	22.8	56.8	16.9	3.5	100
Belgium	23.6	54.5	18.4	3.5	100
Denmark	23.7	56.6	15.8	3.9	100
Finland	24.7	55.5	16.5	3.3	100
France	25.6	53.9	16.9	3.6	100
Germany	21.3	55.7	19.4	3.6	100
Greece	21.8	55.1	19.6	3.5	100
Ireland	30.8	54.1	12.6	2.5	100
Italy	19.8	56.3	20.0	3.9	100
Luxembourg	24.4	56.5	16.0	3.1	100
Netherlands	24.4	57.5	15.0	3.2	100
Portugal	23.5	55.9	17.8	2.8	100
Spain	21.7	56.7	17.9	3.7	100
Sweden	24.2	53.6	17.2	4.9	100
UK	25.3	54.3	16.5	4.0	100
EU-15	23.0	55.4	18.0	3.7	100
Cyprus	31.3	53.4	12.9	2.5	100
Czech Republic	23.4	58.4	15.9	2.3	100
Estonia	25.5	54.2	17.7	2.6	100
Hungary	23.6	56.7	17.2	2.4	100
Latvia	25.3	54.1	18.1	2.5	100
Lithuania	27.1	54.4	16.0	2.5	100
Malta	–	–	–	–	
Poland	28.3	55.2	14.6	1.9	100
Slovak Republic	28.1	56.2	13.5	1.8	100
Slovenia	23.2	57.8	16.8	2.3	100

Source: European Commission (2003)

between different groups of older people are also hidden and this is the reason why these differences are discussed in the second part of the book. A major lacuna in this respect is the absence of data on black and ethnic minority groups.

Demographic ageing is of critical importance in both personal and policy terms and its salience is emphasized by the parallel transformation taking place in the experience and meaning of old age. Retirement is no longer the clear entry point to 'old age' that it once was and, therefore, is anachronistic as a definition of who 'older people' are. More and more people throughout the EU are leaving the labour force in different ways: early retirement, partial retirement, redundancy, unemployment, disability and so on. At the same time, for the reasons outlined above, people are living longer and healthier old ages and, as a result, the threshold of frailty is being pushed back. Thus the interlinked changes in age structure, health and patterns of employment are transforming the nature and experience of old age. They are posing sharp questions about both the traditional, essentially passive roles expected of older people and the extent to which policy makers and major economic and political institutions have adjusted to the fundamental implications of these socio-demographic changes. For example, although European governments have begun to develop policies to promote 'active ageing' the main driving force has been the slump in labour force participation among older workers rather than an understanding of the far-reaching developments taking place in the meaning and experience of ageing (Walker 2002). Some gerontologists, in contrast, have projected a new cultural identity on to these changes in ageing and have downplayed enduring structural divisions based on gender, class and race (Gilleard and Higgs 2001). A wider range of lifestyles is undoubtedly open to today's older people than previous generations, but they are not available to everyone and those in poor health and with low incomes, or those with caring responsibilities, all overwhelmingly women, are excluded (Ginn and Arber 1995). The key issues remain the roles that older people want to play in twenty-first century European societies and how policy makers can ensure that their opportunities are maximized and that social exclusion is minimized.

Definition and measurement of quality of life

Quality of life is a difficult concept to pin down precisely. This is hardly surprising in view of the fact that it is an amalgamation of two equally contested concepts: quality and life. With regard to 'quality' it is reasonable to ask what quality and whose quality? With regard to 'life', the question of what it means, the whole of life or some specified parts of it, immediately confronts those attempting to measure QoL.

With regard to QoL in old age there is a tradition of gerontological research on 'successful ageing', 'positive ageing' and 'healthy ageing' (Baltes 1993; Johnson 1995; Rowe and Kahn 1997). Researchers and practitioners working within this tradition frequently employ a range of health-related indicators as proxies for QoL – functional capacity, health status, psychological wellbeing, social support, morale, dependence, coping and adjustment – without reference to the ways in which older people in general, or specific groups of older people or service users, define their own QoL or the value they place on the different components used by the 'experts'. Furthermore, the dominant scientific and professional approach to assessing QoL in old age has tended to homogenize older people rather than recognising diversity and differences based, for example, on age, gender, race and ethnicity, and disability. Also inherent in this paradigm is a conception of older age as a distinct phase of the life course, one that is detached from middle age and earlier phases (Gubrium and Lynott 1983; Bond 1999). It is not surprising, therefore, that this paradigm is associated with the idea of old age as a problem, something that must be 'adjusted' to. As with general QoL measures it is common for those applied to old age to focus only on health-related quality of life (HRQoL) and to overlook other important aspects.

Recent developments in QoL research are pointing towards the emergence of more holistic and theoretically coherent approaches than those applied previously. First of all there are important, related strands of research, mainly in Europe, aimed at producing both social indicators and theoretically grounded concepts on which to base the measurement of QoL and other related concepts. Two key elements of this European research may be highlighted briefly. On the one hand there is the social-indicator focused research, led by the EU Reporting group (Berger-Schmitt and Jankowitsch 1999; Noll 2000) and Euromodule (Delhey *et al.* 2001), which aim to produce comprehensive lists of indicators for the purposes of social monitoring and reporting. Noll (2000) distinguishes between measures of QoL and quality of society although the indicators he proposes contain elements of both. On the other hand there is the social quality initiative, which has both QoL and quality of society elements together with a focus on social processes (Beck, Van der Maesen and Walker 1997; Beck, Van der Maesen, Thomése and Walker 2001). In the social quality approach it is the nature of the societal processes creating outcomes that are critical as well as the outcomes themselves. The concept emphasises processes of self-realisation and the formation of collective identities as a fundamental dialectic and this underlines the potential role of individual actors within those processes. The level of social quality depends on socio-economic security, social inclusion, social cohesion and social empowerment.

Secondly, phenomenological approaches start with individuals and identify important domains in their lives. For example, the Schedule for the Evaluation of Individual Quality of Life (SEIQoL) seeks from respondents those aspects of life that are considered crucial to their overall QoL (O'Boyle *et al.* 1993). In the SEIQoL the meaning of QoL is determined by the individual, whereas, in contrast, the normative measure of HRQoL reflects the judgement of the researchers. Although the SEIQoL has methodological defects (Bond 1999) it represents an attempt to measure QoL from an individual perspective. Within the ageing field two parallel approaches to assessing QoL from the perspective of older people themselves have been developed. On the one hand, from life-span development psychology, there are attempts to understand subjective meanings of QoL within the context of a person's whole life history (Johnson 1976; Gubrium and Lynott 1983). On the other, QoL has been operationalized recently as a multidimensional phenomenon (Grundy and Bowling 1999; Bowling *et al.* 2002).

Thirdly, within the ageing field, particularly in social gerontology, the critical perspective to understanding old age has influenced research in this field (Phillipson and Walker 1986, 1987; Minkler and Estes 1999; Walker 1999). According to this critical perspective old age is socially constructed and this has three important implications for QoL research. First, contrary to popular stereotypes, the definitions of good QoL for older people are often similar to those for other age groups (Bond 1999), although health and functional capacity figure more strongly, particularly in advanced old age. Second, as human subjects, older people have a right to determine their own meaning of QoL. This means that they should be at the centre of the process of measuring and defining QoL. Third, QoL in old age is influenced as much by social and economic factors as by individual and biological characteristics (Walker 1981). This emphasizes the crucial importance of social structure and culture – race, gender, social class – in determining older people's life experiences and their expectations about what is a good or bad QoL.

At the European level, the Ageing Well project is an ambitious attempt at estimating the direct causal contribution of five key components of QoL (physical health and functioning, mental efficacy, life activity, material security and social support) to the outcome variable 'ageing well'. By definition QoL or wellbeing is a multidimensional concept and, in this case, the validity of the separate domains is derived from previous scientific research rather than subjective opinions. The outcomes of this important comparative work are only just becoming available and are referred to in Chapters 3 and 8.

How are these scientific developments reflected in the five countries represented in this research? With the partial exception of Italy, there are similar trends and scientific debates about the definition and measurement of QoL. HRQoL dominates current approaches to QoL in old age in all of the countries but there are considerable variations in the level of development of research in this topic, especially in the integration of different perspectives, and little or no agreement on the precise way of measuring QoL.

Chapter 2 suggests that there is consensus in Germany on the definition of QoL as a multidimensional welfare term signifying good objective living conditions, a high degree of subjective wellbeing and also collective welfare and the individual satisfaction of needs. This represents an amalgamation of QoL and quality of society approaches. However, when it comes to the questions of how to measure QoL and which components will be included, the consensus breaks down. In the other countries there is nothing like this sort of agreement but, in the two countries with the most developed systems of social reporting, the Netherlands and Sweden, there is perhaps also a generalized acceptance of the range of indicators that constitute QoL.

In Sweden there is a long tradition of social reporting using social indicators, dating from the early 1970s, and an annual population survey focuses on objective living conditions. In the Netherlands the government Social Cultural Planning Office has developed a sophisticated QoL model, including causal relationships – the life situation index (see p. 86). Italy has seen the recent emergence of a more integrated approach to QoL – combining material, environmental, relational and individual factors – which is used to rate QoL in different regions but, as yet, it has not been applied to subgroups such as older people. The UK has a long record of official surveys and public opinion polls but it is only recently that concerted attempts have been made to define the parameters of QoL. However, there is no consensus on the components that should be included.

With regard to measuring QoL, in all five countries it is clear that the tension between objective and subjective approaches is ever present. It is equally clear that, in practice, it is the so-called objective measures that are used most frequently. For example, in Chapter 5 Andersson uses Veenhoven's 'utility of life' quadrant to classify the prevailing approaches to QoL in Swedish gerontology and the majority are concerned with the objective condition of 'livability'. For Italy, Lamura emphasizes the prevalence of economic measures of QoL (per capita income, relative poverty) and objective health-related measures (Chapter 3). Chapter 4 distinguishes not only objective and subjective perspectives in understanding and measuring QoL in the Netherlands but also adds a third, interactive approach, which, with echoes of the social quality method, assesses the degree of fit between the person and his or her environment.

Four of the countries surveyed have substantial experience in measuring QoL in old age. In Italy, however, such measures are not well developed and there is a tendency still to regard older people as one large undifferentiated age group. Germany, Sweden and the UK appear to be the countries in which QoL measures for use with older people have been developed the furthest. Both Sweden and the UK have numerous scientific studies on this topic. In Germany there are three different approaches to the assessment of QoL in old age depending on scientific discipline and how old age is defined.

In Chapter 4 Peters, Bouwman and Knipscheer report that there is very little that is specifically Dutch about the QoL measures used in gerontology, they are mostly adapted from other countries such as the US and the UK. For example, the SEIQoL has been adapted specifically for use in the Netherlands. The most frequently used measures of QoL in all five countries are predetermined instruments. The UK is distinctive in having developed an individual older person's perspective on measuring QoL. This has been progressed furthest by Bowling and her colleagues (2002) and Gabriel and Bowling (2004) under the GO Programme (Chapter 6).

Environments of ageing

Housing is a very important aspect of the QoL of older people everywhere. In Western Europe it is usually a place associated with individual and family biographies and, therefore, is imbued with meaning and aspects of identity. It is also the location where older people spend much of their time and the proportion of time spent at home rises in old age. For example, in Germany, the Berlin Ageing Study shows that, between the ages of 70 and 103, 80 per cent of activities are carried out within a person's home. In Sweden older people spend 80 to 85 per cent of the day at home.

In the five countries and across the EU as a whole there is a clear trend towards living alone in old age, a trend that is particularly marked in advanced old age. Table 1.3 shows that by 2050, in the EU-15 countries, nearly one-third of people aged 65 and over will be living alone and, among those aged 80 and over, it will be more than two-fifths. The variation between countries is significant and appears to follow a north/south pattern (cf Walker 1993) in which the Nordic member states have relatively high levels of single-housing occupation and the southern states low ones. Sweden, as the representative of the three Nordic countries in this book, has above average predicted rates for older people living alone in 2010; Italy, representing the four southern countries in the EU-15, has below average predicted rates. As is explained more fully later in this chapter and discussed in Chapter 3, with regard to Italy, the increase in the proportion of older people living alone in Europe is not, by itself, indicative of greater isolation. In fact it reflects a preference for separate dwellings that varies between countries and is not necessarily held with equal strength by younger and older generations. In advanced old age, living alone is a highly gendered experience: for example in Sweden today, among those aged 80 and over, the proportion of women living alone (81 per cent) is nearly twice that of men (42 per cent).

The five countries surveyed display a wide range of experience with regard to the quality of housing. At one end, in Sweden, the housing conditions enjoyed by older people do not differ markedly from those of the general population, although it is estimated that some 12 per cent of households aged 45 and over living in apartments do not have access to a lift. At the other end, in Italy, the housing conditions of older people are lower than the national average, particularly among those aged 75 and over. Therefore, lack of basic housing security is a key factor in Italy in diminishing the QoL of older people: 68 per cent of older person households have no lift and 24 per cent lack an effective heating system. In Italy, those over 75 often suffer from multiple disadvantage: living alone with low incomes and restricted personal autonomy. Not surprisingly there is a high incidence of domestic accidents among older people, with those aged 65 and over representing 26 per cent of the victims of such accidents and 76 per cent of the casualties resulting from domestic accidents.

The Netherlands, Germany and the UK are ranged between these two extremes in that order. The Netherlands has seen a recent improvement in the quality of housing among older people as a result of an increase in purpose-built housing and in the space occupied by older people in residential care homes. Chapter 2 notes significant differences in German older people's housing quality between the eastern and western parts. In the UK, older people's housing quality is lower than the average and, especially among the very elderly, is often in a poor state of repair.

Table 1.3 Residential status of older people, 2010 (%)

Country	Age group	Living alone	Living with a partner	Older households	Institutions
Austria	65+	31	52	13	4
	80+	43	29	17	11
Belgium	65+	35	48	13	4
	80+	51	28	14	8
Denmark	65+	42	52	2	5
	80+	62	26	2	10
Finland	65+	38	48	9	5
	80+	49	23	14	14
France	65+	34	54	6	5
	80+	46	34	10	10
Germany	65+	35	56	5	3
	80+	52	29	9	10
Greece	65+	27	57	10	6
	80+	36	35	16	12
Ireland	65+	32	42	17	9
	80+	39	19	23	19
Italy	65+	27	52	14	7
	80+	39	30	17	13
Luxembourg	65+	28	52	16	4
	80+	38	28	25	9
Netherlands	65+	33	55	3	9
	80+	44	27	5	24
Portugal	65+	23	57	18	2
	80+	32	35	30	4
Spain	65+	22	58	18	2
	80+	30	34	32	4
Sweden	65+	42	54	2	2
	80+	62	30	3	4
UK	65+	35	52	8	4
	80+	50	31	11	8
EU-15	65+	32	54	9	4
	80+	45	31	14	10

Source: European Commission (2003)

It is obvious that when older people are in some form of institutional care their QoL is dominated by their residential environment and its regime. The Netherlands has the highest proportion of older people in such care within the EU-15 (Table 1.4) and research indicates relatively high levels of personal satisfaction. One reason for this is the recent increase in the space allocation in residential care homes resulting from new purpose-built accommodation. There is much less satisfaction among older people in nursing homes where single rooms are rare. In contrast, in Italy the residential care environment is poor and older people are able to exercise very little personal autonomy.

Chapters 2 to 6 suggest higher than average levels of satisfaction among older people with their residential environment in the five countries but less so with regard to access to local amenities, especially transport (see below). Older people clearly use multiple criteria in assessing the quality of their neighbourhood and, in Germany, the key issues are a 'good' neighbourhood, quiet surroundings, good environmental conditions and transport. In Sweden nine out of ten older people consider proximity to public transport and domiciliary services as the most important issues. Also eight out of ten older people in Sweden consider it important to live with people of all ages.

Apart from transport the major area of dissatisfaction concerns personal safety and particularly the fear of being alone on a street at night. It seems that these fears, particularly among very elderly women, are found in all five countries and are having a negative impact on QoL in old age. It is well known that such perceived insecurity is related to age, location (rural/urban) and neighbourhood. Although fears concerning personal safety rise with age, paradoxically, older people are less likely than younger ones to be the victims of personal attacks (partly because they go out less often).

Turning to transport, which is widely acknowledged as an important but under-researched contributor to QoL in old age, Chapters 2 to 6 reveal significant differences between countries in access to and satisfaction with transport. For those that have one, the car is the preferred method of transport (older people with cars use them for most journeys in Italy, the Netherlands and the UK) and buses are the most common form of public transport. The high importance given to transport by older people in Sweden has already been noted and this appears to be true for the other countries except Italy, where it is not regarded as a major QoL issue. Older Italians are generally satisfied with public transport, apart from the cost. In contrast, in the UK, one-third of people aged 60 and over have one or more activities that they are unable to do as often as they would like because of lack of transport. The Netherlands and Sweden have gone further than other countries to develop public transport schemes catering especially for older people. For example, the Netherlands has a system of collective transport entitlements and 75 per cent of new beneficiaries over-65.

Information and communications technology (ICT) is widely seen as having the potential to substantially improve the QoL of older people (ETAN 1998), however, the current position in the five countries suggests not only that this potential is far from being realized but also that the familiar barriers to takeup still remain. One-fifth of people aged 65 to 84 have access to a home computer in Sweden, compared with 15 per cent among over-65s in Italy. In the Netherlands almost one-half of older people experience difficulties in using equipment or machines and they also have lower ownership of ICT products than among younger people (lowest among those aged 75 and over). Older people are one of the most disadvantaged groups in the information society and are also disadvantaged by non-inclusive product design.

Physical and mental health

This has been a major focus for gerontological research for several decades and there is a well-established association between chronic illness and disability and advanced old age. Not surprisingly, therefore, the country chapters in Part I do not reveal major differences in either the research agendas or the findings from research in this area. There is similar agreement that health is a major determinant of QoL. For example, 97 per cent of people in the 40 to 85 age group surveyed in Germany said that good health is one of their most important life goals and this centrality of health increases during the second half of life.

The most common chronic conditions in old age are lung disease, heart and cardiovascular diseases, diabetes, stroke, joint disorders, dementia, depression and impaired vision and hearing. The health complaints that have the strongest impact on daily living – the 'geriatric giants' – are mental/cognitive functioning, mobility, balance and stability, vision and hearing and incontinence. Although a great deal of research and policy attention has been rightly given to the chronic mental condition of dementia – the prevalence of which increases in old age and which places major demands on both paid and unpaid carers as well as healthcare systems – the prevalence of anxiety and depression in old age is around two to three times higher. The main mental health conditions – anxiety, depression and cognitive disorder (including dementia) – have a substantial impact on medical services.

Chapters 2 to 6 remind us that gerontological research has repeatedly demonstrated that there is a gap between objectively assessed health and condition and self-perceptions. Many older people say they are in good health when they are suffering from one or more chronic conditions – the 'selective optimization with compensation' observation (Baltes and Baltes 1996). This emphasizes the great importance of looking beyond medical criteria in assessing QoL. Quality of life is also influenced critically by people's subjective appraisal of their own health status. Research points to the importance of subjective health status in determining how older people regard the ageing process. Subjectively perceived health is also a sensitive indicator of mortality as well as of the use of healthcare services.

Chapters 2 to 6 all report a general improvement in self-reported health in old age over the last few decades but no corresponding reduction in the prevalence of chronic illness and disability, nor in the takeup of medical services. In all countries there is a continuing gender disparity in late old age, with women being much more likely than men to experience chronic physical and mental conditions. For example in the UK, nearly one-half of women aged 85 and over are unable to walk in the street unaided compared with less than one-fifth of men. Swedish data questions the 'compression of morbidity' thesis by showing that, over the last 20 years, there has been 0.2 more years with full health for both sexes between the ages of 65 and 84. The number of years with impaired health increased by 2.1 years for men and 1.6 years for women in the same age group.

Employment and retirement

Retirement has been a central aspect of ageing research for more than half a century but it is only recently that employment has become a major focus of attention. This recent interest stems mainly from the realization that population ageing means workforce ageing and the focus, among policy makers, especially in the EU countries, is the paradox of increasing longevity coupled with declining economic activity (Walker 1997). Employment is a key determinant of QoL in old age in the sense that it has a large influence on the amount of pension a person receives and the other resources at their command and, therefore, is an important determinant of their general economic status. There is also research evidence on the importance of work for identity and inner as well as outer need satisfaction. However, there is no evidence that the absence of employment *necessarily* affects QoL in old age in a substantial way, although recent UK research shows that compared with other groups in the third age (50 to 74) those in employment *after* pension age have the highest levels of life satisfaction (Chapter 5).

First of all retirement is not associated with a decline in health status (unless, of course, poor health precipitated it). Indeed, Swedish research indicates that there is a significant, if short-term, health gain – the so-called 'retirement dip' – whereby, particularly for white-collar workers, it is not until four years after retirement that the proportion reporting long-term illness rises again. For both men and women the incidence of fatigue is lowest around retirement. Secondly, German longitudinal research indicates that the transition to retirement cannot be regarded as a reduction in QoL. It is undeniable that retirement entails losses, for example in social status, finance and network satisfaction. However, older people are able to compensate for some of these losses, for example by replacing social relations in employment with other social contacts. According to Reichert and Weidekamp-Maicher the key factors influencing positive wellbeing in retirement are:

◆ a positive attitude towards entering retirement;

◆ a high degree of satisfaction with achievements in previous employment;

◆ a transition free from conflicts and entirely voluntary;

◆ a high level of wellbeing *before* retirement (optimism, emotional stability and a positive view of old age) which is a predictor of subjective wellbeing *after* retirement.

There is also some research evidence that subjective evaluations of retirement depend on societal attitudes towards it (Chapter 2).

The five country chapters in Part I also reveal important differences in the retirement experience. For example with regard to occupational class (Sweden): although there is some levelling of health differences, some are maintained and there is a delayed emergence of differences. In Germany there are important variations in retirement between the new and old federal states. Older employees in the east are more likely to be threatened with or affected by unemployment, which results in low income and loss of esteem (loss of work is felt particularly acutely in the east). There are also gender differences with women reaping the results of disadvantages experienced in the middle phase of life resulting, for example, in lower incomes in old age. Women tend to leave employment in a less standard way than men.

For people in their 50s employment and age discrimination are key issues. This is true in all five countries and in the EU-15 as a whole (Table 1.4). Low employment rates among people aged 50 and over also reflect a number of factors, including the previous policy era in most EU countries in which older workers were encouraged to leave the labour market (Kohli *et al.* 1991; Walker 1997). Thus the very low employment rate among those over 50 in Italy results from the policy, negotiated by trades unions, which allowed widespread early exit – in the case of the public sector 'baby pensions' were provided after only 15 or 16 years of work for women and 20 or 21 years for men. It is partly as a result of this mass early exit that Italy is witnessing the emergence of second careers, with 7 to 8 per cent of the total retired population (18 per cent of the 50 to 64 age group) continuing to work. Research in the UK emphasizes the negative psychological impact of involuntary job loss and unemployment on

Table 1.4 Employment rates in the Third Age, 2000

	50–54	55–59	60–64	65–69	70–74
Austria	72.1	42.4	12.1	5.5	2.8
Belgium	61.0	37.9	12.4	2.3	1.8
Denmark	80.8	72.6	30.9	8.1	–
Finland	80.1	58.5	22.8	5.0	2.9
France	74.9	48.1	10.2	2.1	0.9
Germany	74.3	56.4	19.6	4.9	2.3
Greece	61.8	48.2	31.3	11.2	3.7
Ireland	64.4	53.1	35.8	14.7	2.7
Italy	58.1	36.5	18.0	6.0	2.7
Luxembourg	66.4	38.9	14.5	3.4	–
Netherlands	71.4	54.1	18.5	5.1	2.9
Portugal	71.9	58.3	45.2	27.1	18.8
Spain	58.4	46.0	26.4	3.9	1.0
Sweden	83.8	78.6	46.0	14.2	5.6
UK	76.1	63.2	36.1	11.3	4.8
EU-15	70.0	51.9	22.6	6.5	2.9

Source: European Commission (2003)

17

older workers and the fact that this lessens as one approaches pension age. This research also documents exclusion from training and the negative stereotypes held by many employers. In the five countries under comparison here (and in the whole EU-15) Sweden is the opposite pole to Italy, with the highest employment rate among older people. Influential factors here are anti-discrimination measures, occupational health services and active employment policies.

Income and wealth

It is self-evident that income is a fundamental contributor to wellbeing and QoL. There is a positive relationship between income and participation at all adult ages (Townsend 1979) and also, in old age, with objective and subjective health and wellbeing and the experience of ageing. Conversely research also demonstrates the negative impact of low incomes on mortality, morbidity and social participation (Wilkinson 1999). Differences in income in old age are determined mainly in earlier years including at birth, particularly by employment status and, if employed, type of employment, gender and race.

All five countries report recent improvements in the living standards of older people (due to some extent to public policy) but the differences between the member states in the levels of income received by pensioners and, in particular, their likelihood of experiencing poverty, observed in the early 1990s (Walker, Guillemard and Alber 1993) still persist. In view of the importance of public pensions in the EU such cross-national differences reflect, to some extent, the level of spending on pensions by the member states, with Germany (13.0 per cent), Italy (15.1 per cent) and the Netherlands (13.3 per cent) all being above EU average spenders on pensions (as a percentage of GDP in 1999) with Sweden (12.2 per cent) and the UK (11.5 per cent) being below the average (12.7 per cent). Of course such data should take account of the varying size of the older (65 plus) population in these EU countries – which ranges from 13.1 million in Germany to 2.2 million in the Netherlands.

Of the countries surveyed the UK has the highest proportion of older people living on low incomes, despite the recent improvement in their living standards – one in four pensioner families are in the bottom fifth of the income distribution. In comparative terms it has by far the highest proportion of older people at risk of poverty, particularly in relation to other northern EU countries (Table 1.5). At the same time, in the UK, there are increasing numbers of relatively affluent older people, which has led to the assessment that there are 'two nations' in old age. In contrast, in Italy, while there is some risk of poverty among the retired, particularly among very elderly lone women, the income distribution between different age groups is more balanced than in other EU countries and this results in a lower poverty rate in old age than in Germany and the UK. A key factor here is the redistributive role of the family through which income flows between the generations. There is also a high propensity to save in Italy. Sweden has the lowest level of poverty among people aged 50 and over in these five countries and, indeed, in the whole of the EU. The Netherlands has the lowest poverty rate among both those over the age of 65 and the retired.

Table 1.5 EU Poverty Rates,[1] 1998

	Age group		
	50–64	**65+**	**Retired**
Austria	10	21	14
Belgium	16	20	17
Denmark	4	27	23
Finland	6	8	7
France	15	18	16
Germany	13	13	14
Greece	22	36	36
Ireland	12	24	20
Italy	17	16	13
Luxembourg	10	9	11
Netherlands	6	6	3
Portugal	17	34	28
Spain	17	14	12
Sweden	4	7	–
UK	13	40	38
EU-15	14	20	18

Note: 1. 60% of median equivalized income
Source: European Commission (2003)

The longstanding observation that poverty and low incomes are concentrated in late old age and particularly among lone older women (Walker, Guillemard and Alber 1993) is confirmed by Chapters 2 to 6. The EU's globally superior pension systems have not succeeded in ending gender inequalities in old age and, in some cases, may have reinforced them.

Family and support networks

The five country chapters in Part II on participation and social support begin by reporting the current knowledge about family and support networks. It is acknowledged widely that personal relationships are important for wellbeing and that intergenerational family solidarity is a critical determinant of QoL in old age. The chapters reveal differences in the role of the family on the expected north-south axis, although the Italian case indicates that the 'southern European model' is changing. In the northern countries there has been a major increase in older people living alone in the past two decades whereas, in Italy, despite a doubling of the numbers living alone in this period, a relatively low proportion of older people are in this situation – less than one in four compared with one in three in Germany and the UK (projections shown in Table 1.3). In contrast to the northern countries, the family in Italy is overwhelmingly the main source of support in terms of social contacts as well as the provision of care. Extended family relationships also appear to be more complex than in the other countries and less importance is attached to friends. In northern countries the family is still central in the lives of older people but its role is changing and friends play an important part in providing assistance and support.

Research demonstrates that having a confidante, such as a partner or friend, is a key element in social relationships and support. Dutch surveys show that older people living with a partner have more relationships and more support exchanges than those who live alone. On the other hand, older people living alone have more neighbours and friends in their support networks compared to those living with others (Chapter 9). Relationships and personal support decline in late old age.

European research has previously shown the high levels of social contact between older people and their families, despite the growth of residential separation (Walker 1993; Walker and Maltby 1997) and Chapters 7 to 11 also emphasize this 'intimacy at a distance' (Rosenmayer and Kockeis 1963). For example, pioneering research in the Netherlands on the networks of older people found that over three-quarters of children and 40 per cent of their brothers and sisters (and their partners) were regarded as being part of their network. Recent research on grandparenting in several countries reveals frequent contact between grandparents and their grandchildren, particularly when the latter are young; it also shows a wide diversity in grandparenting styles, and that grandparenting is very important to the psychological wellbeing of older people.

Neighbours and friends are important contributors to QoL in old age: neighbours give more emotional support and less instrumental support than friends, and friends give more instrumental support. Friendships are more important for women than men and, in advanced old age, women tend to have more contacts with friends.

Delving beneath the relatively common studies of the frequency of social contacts, German longitudinal research has shown a relationship between social integration and support and higher life expectancy and QoL. Older people who are more extravert and externally oriented are not only more satisfied with their health but have a higher degree of wellbeing. Critical in the wellbeing associated with networks is not the availability or frequency of contacts but the perceived closeness and informational value of the contacts. German research has also looked at the *negative* impact of relationships – the experience of excessive demands, loss of autonomy, lack of reciprocity, conflicts, abuse and neglect. This shows that older people experience contact with others as a burden if it is emotionally neutral or not meaningful. All this suggests that what matters in social relationships is the meaning older people attach to them. Objective measures are insufficient to connect networks and QoL, research needs to focus on emotional meaning and the maintenance of important values such as reciprocity, autonomy and self-sufficiency.

Participation

It is conventional wisdom in social gerontology and in policy circles that activity is essential for a good QoL. Certainly activity is highly correlated with health in old age. The EU has relatively high rates of social participation in all age groups (European Commission 2001) but, everywhere, participation declines with age, particularly among men. For example, in the Netherlands, 74 per cent of those under 75 are members of organizations compared with 50 per cent of the over-75s. Sweden and the Netherlands report particularly high levels of participation in organizations and associations, the highest rate being in Sweden – 88 per cent of men and 82 per cent of women aged 65 to 84 – mainly as a result of the high membership of pensioners' organizations in that country. Voluntary activity appears to be high in all countries. However, despite these high levels of participation there is no evidence that those older people conforming to the stereotype of 'active' old age are anything more than a small minority. Research is lacking on the association between participation and QoL in old age.

Recently research has begun to explore the meaning and experience of acute exclusion in the form of loneliness. For example, in the UK a recent study has shown that loneliness in old age has not increased in the last 50 years despite the popular assumption that it has (Victor *et al.* 2003). Extensive research in the Netherlands points to three important facts about loneliness: it means an absence in a person's social relations, it is a feeling that differs from being alone, and it is unpleasant and depressing. Moreover loneliness occurs throughout the lifecourse but increases with age. The most lonely are not necessarily the oldest people but those with limited resources in terms of relationships and/or health. Thus loneliness is not related to ageing as such but to changes associated with age, such as the loss of a partner, a limited social network, infrequent contacts and poor health. Key indicators of loneliness are: the loss of a partner; gender (men without partners are more likely to be lonely than women); socio-economic status (those with high levels of income and education have the widest networks); a relationship based on mutual trust (having one or more people to trust reduces the chances of loneliness); and living alone in advanced old age.

Services and quality of life

Older people are the main users of health and social care services and, therefore, the quality of those services can have a critical bearing on their QoL. (Social security also has a major influence on QoL in old age but here we are concentrating on the personal services.) It is clear that health and social services are in flux in all five countries as well as there being substantial variations in the availability of such services for older people between different EU countries, particularly on the north/south axis (Walker, Guillemard and Alber 1993; Walker and Maltby 1997; Pacolet and Bouten 2000). Thus Italy has a far lower level of social services than the other countries, although in all five of them there are variations in the availability of such services between municipalities.

In the Netherlands there is a new policy emphasis on the modernization of social care services for older people, primarily in response to their desire for greater independence. Key themes in this process are accessibility and suitability of the care services. Overall government policy is aimed at encouraging independent living. A new form of care funding is individualized budgets – the person allocated budgets – which provide cash in place of in-kind care. The continuation of official efforts to improve the quality of care is indicated by the fall in the number of multi-person rooms in nursing homes. The Dutch research evidence suggests that older people in nursing homes want privacy, a reduction in waiting times following the use of the alarm button, freedom in deciding when to go to the toilet and when to get up, and being able to hold confidential conversations, and that these are the aspects of QoL that could be improved.

German researchers have only recently shifted their focus from 'objective' QoL assessments, with respect to older people receiving nursing care, towards subjective assessments such as satisfaction and wellbeing. Ensuring the best quality of care is not an explicit goal of the statutory nursing care insurance but it is a major issue of current debate in Germany and, particularly, a debate about what measures are suitable for ensuring quality of nursing care. There is very little systematic research on this topic. As in the UK there has been a recent emergence of the perspective of nursing care service users and patient satisfaction measures are being used, however, there is a lack of research on subjective wellbeing. Again, as in the UK, assessments of QoL in nursing care reveal clear differences in the criteria used to evaluate it between patients and professionals: the former emphasize wellbeing and the latter the quality of nursing.

Research in the UK has shown the importance of low intensity support for older people to enable them to live in their own homes and the underdevelopment of preventative activities – a longstanding finding (Walker 1982a, 1982b). Yet, in both the UK and Sweden, there has been a concentration of home care on the most severely disabled in the last decade. Research in the UK also shows an important connection between identity and older people's perception of independence (Baldock and Hadlow 2002). The recent introduction of a National Service Framework for Older People recognizes the lack of consistency in service provision in the UK and the existence of age discrimination in the health and social services.

Life satisfaction and wellbeing

Life satisfaction has been described as the subjective expression of QoL (Fernández-Ballesteros *et al.* 2002: 25) and is commonly seen in gerontological circles as an indicator of successful ageing (Freund and Baltes 1998). The five countries in this book emphasize the previously observed internal differences between EU countries in attitudes towards key areas of life quality (Walker 1993; Walker and Maltby 1997). They also underline the long acknowledged gap between 'objective' and subjective living conditions and the importance of both health and subjective wellbeing to QoL in old age.

In the Netherlands most older people feel happy, though the percentage declines with age: nearly half are satisfied with the lives they lead and roughly one-sixth are downright dissatisfied with life. The main sources of variation with age are that, in advanced old age, people more frequently suffer from health problems or live alone. Older people assess their own health more positively than is justified by 'objective' criteria and older people judge their health to be poor more often than younger people, but this seems to plateau at around the age of 75. Residents of nursing homes or sheltered housing assess their own health more negatively than those living independently.

German research in this area has produced inconsistent findings. Some studies show that subjective QoL increases with age while some indicate the opposite. Very elderly people experience a high level of wellbeing in spite of losses and limitations: 87 per cent of those over 70 in West Germany and 82 per cent in East Germany report feeling very or fairly happy. The Berlin Ageing Study paints a positive picture of wellbeing in old age – the majority (63 per cent) of 70 to 103 year olds are satisfied with their past and present life. But, with increasing age there is a decrease in positive emotions and in the anticipation of future life satisfaction in old age because cross-sectional surveys show that older people have higher levels of satisfaction than younger age groups. This suggests high levels of adaptability and resilience but, also, the danger that they will not take advantage of opportunities if they need to or that the policy system will not be as responsive as it might be. Coping strategies are shown to be an essential mechanism for safeguarding wellbeing in old age (for example in response to loss).

Research in the UK also reveals relatively high levels of life satisfaction among older people, with no major differences between this group and the middle aged. When older people are asked to prioritize QoL domains, people over 75 are more likely than young people to select their own health and ability to get about and less likely to choose relationships with families, other relatives, finances and employment.

In Italy it is family relationships that are the most important source of life satisfaction among older people, regardless of age or gender, and health and financial situation that causes the highest dissatisfaction. Some four out of five older people are completely or quite satisfied with their present life. Various Italian studies point to the centrality of health-related issues in the QoL of older people.

Swedish research adds to this picture of general satisfaction and the key role of health status (objective and subjective) in two important ways. First, it emphasizes the significance of biographical research in showing that the meaning of old age cannot be separated from the rest of the lifecourse. Second, research on the wellbeing of nonogenarians demonstrates that high life satisfaction is a function of excellent subjective health, good social relations, participation in pleasurable activities and an extraverted and emotionally stable personality. This research also suggests that 'outlook on life', 'social and emotional ties', 'engagement with the outside world' and 'physical capability' are important contributors to subjective wellbeing. In late old age personality is the major determinant of wellbeing.

Although strictly beyond the scope of this five-nation study, important Spanish research of life satisfaction has highlighted the relative contributory importance of different socio-demographic and psychological factors. The theoretical model constructed by Fernández-Ballesteros and her colleagues (2001) explained 69 per cent of the life satisfaction variance (Figure 1.1). Socio-demographic characteristics (educational level and monthly income) are the antecedents of all factors in the model, with direct effects on life satisfaction and indirect effects via psychosocial factors such as activity, physical illness and perceived health. Among the psychosocial factors activity was found to have the strongest impact on life satisfaction (here 'activity' included physical activities, satisfaction with these and social relationships). Also, in common with other research, health – physical illness and subjective health assessment – is seen to be an explanatory variable in life satisfaction.

Future research priorities

Each chapter in Part II makes proposals for further research on QoL in old age, which are summarized here. A striking feature of the research priorities identified is that some research gaps in one country have already been filled in

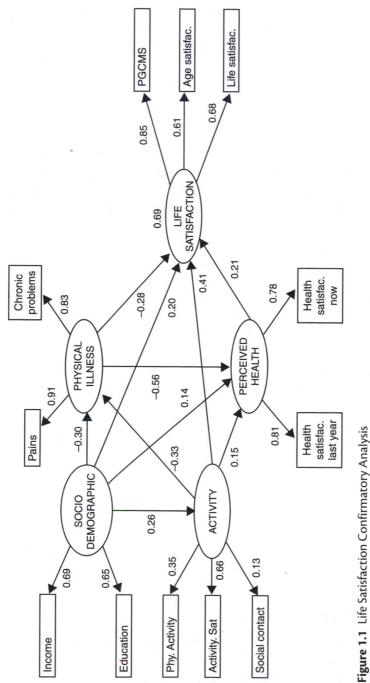

Figure 1.1 Life Satisfaction Confirmatory Analysis

Source: Fernandez-Ballesteros et al. (2001)

another. This suggests that there is considerable scope for sharing research knowledge between EU countries. There is a common need for research in all of the countries in the following eight fields.

Defining and measuring quality of life

The EU needs more standardized measures of QoL in old age (generally) and, especially, ones that move beyond health and physical and mental functioning and recognize the multidimensional nature of the concept. There must be a key role for the EU's Framework Programmes in encouraging such research. An important element of this necessary endeavour is the inclusion of older people's own definitions of QoL. National resources such as the UK's GO programme and Nestor in the Netherlands must be shared more effectively.

Environment, housing and information and communications technology (ICT)

'Ecological gerontology' and 'architectural gerontology' are relatively neglected in the EU (with the exception of Germany) and there is a need for more research on inclusive living and design. Transport is critical to QoL yet is poorly understood. Information and communications technology has a huge potential but poor practice and there is a need for interdisciplinary research on its possible uses and high quality evaluations of ICT applications.

Physical and mental health

This area has dominated research in gerontology and has benefited older people substantially but there is insufficient sharing of information and, especially, data between countries. For example, there are important longitudinal studies in Germany, Italy and Sweden that could be a major resource for research in other countries. There is a need for research on subjective health and how this interacts with other QoL factors. Again older people themselves should be the focus of research: the criteria they use to assess their own physical and mental health and the strategies they employ to maintain their own wellbeing and how effective these are.

Income and wealth

There is a common research gap on QoL differences based on socio-economic security and the relationship between income and wealth and subjectively assessed QoL.

Participation

The concept of 'active ageing' is inconsistently understood in the EU and the relationship between participation and QoL needs further research, including comparative studies.

Services

There should be more comparative evaluations of the impact of services on older people's QoL.

Wellbeing and satisfaction

All countries require a better understanding of older people's definitions of wellbeing and which aspects of life give them satisfaction. This is a topic ripe for comparative analysis.

Ethnicity and migration

There is a major gap in knowledge about ageing and QoL among black and ethnic minorities. This topic has been the focus of much recent research in the UK and efforts should be made to share the findings with other EU countries.

Conclusion

This comparative study has generated a great deal of information about the quality of life in old age and has identified current gaps in knowledge and the need for further research. As well as setting a research agenda it has demonstrated the value of taking stock before undertaking new research. In this process it is clear that there is a considerable amount of duplication of research between even the small group of EU member states represented here. How far this duplication is warranted by national differences in culture, institutions and policy is an open question but what is certain is that there is insufficient pooling of research data by scientists or policy makers in the different member states. It is obvious that an effective approach to sharing research information and priorities across the member states has the potential to add considerable value to the EU's ageing research portfolio.

The chapters in this book provide a comprehensive picture of QoL in old age. A high level of standardization has been achieved across the chapters by face-to-face meetings among the researchers concerned, the first of which agreed the template for the twin country chapters, electronic follow-up contacts and a workshop in London that discussed drafts of the chapters (see www.shef.ac.uk/uni/projects.gop/index.htm). The workshop was attended by a wide range of experts on QoL in old age from nine countries and the chapters were revised in response to the discussion as well as editorial comments.

This book is intended as a European companion to the GO programme and, specifically, the two volumes that report the programme as a whole (Walker and Hagan Hennessy 2004; Walker 2005). Chapters 6 and 11 summarize some of that material but, as Dean (2003) has pointed out, the wealth of information generated by the programme is the 'equivalent of the British Library' in this field, therefore readers are urged to consult the other volumes in this GO series.

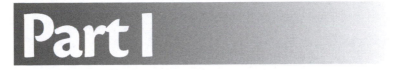

Part I

Quality of life in old age: definitions, environments and socio-economic aspects

2

Germany: quality of life in old age I

Manuela Weidekamp-Maicher and Monika Reichert

Introduction

Research on quality of life (QoL) originates from different research traditions in Germany, each with a different perspective on the term 'quality of life'. In economic and social research QoL is understood in connection with the monitoring of the national welfare system. Viewed historically, welfare was initially equated with material prosperity, and social progress was measured by the increase in the standard of living (Glatzer and Zapf 1984; Glatzer 1998). Since the 1970s, however, 'subjective welfare' has been added to 'objective welfare'. Wellbeing is 'an interpretation of welfare' (Noll 1997) that places special emphasis on the individual. In comparison QoL is a multidimensional concept that includes both the physical and nonphysical, the objective and subjective, individual and collective welfare, and stresses 'better' over 'more' (Noll 1997). The main databases that record objective and subjective social indicators are the Welfare Survey (WS), the Socio-Economic Panel (SOEP) and the German Aging Survey (Kohli and Künemund 2000).[1]

Another tradition is psychologically oriented wellbeing and health research (Becker 1982; Mayring 1987; Abele and Becker 1991; Ravens-Sieberer and Cieza 2000), which places major emphasis on the term 'subjective quality of life'. Psycho-social gerontology has also dealt with the concept of wellbeing by analysing wellbeing and satisfaction as indicators of successful ageing (Baltes 1993).

Quality of life, life satisfaction and wellbeing have seldom been combined into one integrated whole. This is reflected with regard to older people: gerontology has still not produced a theory of QoL in old age. Objective and subjective dimensions of the construct, depending on the particular area of research, can, however, be said to be well researched. In the areas of health, living conditions and the role of social networks and social support in old age, particularly good progress is being made in measuring objective and subjective QoL. This is also true for the state of knowledge in relation to the significance of various indicators of socio-economic status. Research in relation to the very old, however, is lacking in most dimensions of QoL and this is likely to become one of the greatest challenges for future gerontological research (Lehr 2000).

Quality of life: definitions, measurement and the role of policy

According to Glatzer and Zapf (1984) QoL represents a 'multi-dimensional welfare term that signifies good "objective" living conditions and a high degree of "subjective" wellbeing, and also includes collective welfare in addition to the individual satisfaction of needs' (Glatzer and Zapf 1984; Noll 1997; Glatzer 1998: 428). Quality of life, then, contains two dimensions: an assessment of the living situation based on 'objective' indicators, as well as an individual perception or interpretation of this situation which is an expression of subjective QoL. Perceived QoL is equated with the term 'subjective wellbeing', which has emotional, cognitive and evaluative aspects. The focus can be life in general or specific dimensions including private and public dimensions (Delhey and Böhnke 1999). Quality of life includes not only all the individually important areas of life, but also nonmaterial and collective values such as liberty, justice, protection of the natural environment, and responsibility for future generations (Zapf 1984; Noll 1997; Glatzer 1998).

While there is wide acceptance of the general definition of QoL its component parts are conceptualized quite differently. Differences exist mainly in the definition and measurement of subjective QoL. While Glatzer and Zapf distinguish merely between a cognitively oriented component of 'satisfaction' and an emotional component of 'happiness' with reference to subjective wellbeing, Mayring (1987: 371), following Lawton (1984, quoted in Mayring 1987: 371; Mayring 1991: 51), assumes four aspects of subjective QoL: a negative emotional factor (negative affect); a positive emotional factor (positive affect); happiness as the conviction that the positive emotions are long-term; and goal congruence: the conviction of having reached one's own goals.

Happiness represents the most comprehensive wellbeing factor and involves both current (state) and habitual wellbeing (trait). Current wellbeing includes the temporary experience of a person, positive emotions, moods and bodily sensations, as well as the absence of worries and complaints (Becker 1991: 13). Habitual wellbeing means 'statements about wellbeing that are typical for a person, i.e., judgments about aggregated emotional experiences' (Becker 1991: 15).

Measuring QoL

There is little agreement as to how to measure QoL. This is especially the case with subjective QoL. The questions of whether subjective QoL, measured by the individual's subjective sense of satisfaction with life, is a dependent variable of objective life conditions, in which causal direction they stand to each other and what the appropriate indices are for subjective wellbeing and its correlates, have often been discussed but remain unresolved. Thus, statements about wellbeing in gerontology are frequently assessed as indices of the effectiveness of social policy, medical or psychiatric interventions. A high degree of satisfaction with life is understood as an indication of 'successful ageing' (Thomae 1987; Baltes and Baltes 1992; Baltes 1993), 'successful' adjustment to retirement (Mayring 2000) or as the success of coping strategies (Rothermund *et al.* 1994; Rothermund and Brandstädter 1998).

The individual disciplines are distinct in the measures they use:

- Answers to individual questions (for example the Welfare Survey) or multiple items and scales (the German Ageing Survey).

- Scales that were especially developed for healthy, infirm or demented older people or scales for general sample surveys.

- Instruments that record the emotional or cognitive components of wellbeing – or a combination of both, for example the German version of PANAS (Positive and Negative Affect Schedule, Krohne *et al.* 1996); the SWLS (Satisfaction with Life Scale, Schumacher *et al.* 2003); and the ABS (Affect Balance Scale, Becker 1982).

Assessment of the emotional components of wellbeing inquire about the frequency of positive and negative feelings. Cognitively oriented measurement instruments concentrate on the assessment of the contents of life and satisfaction with life. Some researchers have introduced further dimensions into the measurement, such as adjustment, coping, attitude towards life and spiritual health. In addition to these problems of dimensionality and the relative weighting of individual aspects, there is a continuing debate about the links between subjective and objective indicators (Abele and Becker 1991; Brandtstädter and Greve 1992; Bulmahn 1996).

Environments of ageing

Living conditions designed to meet people's needs in terms of spatial, infrastructural and technological environment have considerable significance for QoL in old age (Bundesministerium für Familie, Senioren, Frauen und Jugend [BMFSFJ] 2001a: 41). There has been proven success by ecological-gerontological research in analysing not only the living area but also the residential surroundings including new technologies as resources in old age (Wahl *et al.* 1999).

Living conditions

The contribution of the living environment to QoL in old age is mainly via its support for independent living in spite of the loss of health. This contribution is emphasized by the results of time-use analyses showing that the portion of time spent within one's own home climbs continually for both sexes after the age of 55. Compared with younger people, older people not only spend more time within their own homes but leisure interests and activities are also more heavily concentrated on the inner home area or the immediate residential surroundings (Küster 1998). In the Berlin Ageing Study, those surveyed aged 70 to 103 years indicated that they performed 80 per cent of their activities in their own home (Baltes, Maas *et al.* 1996). Independence in living, health, cognitive activity and performance, social activity and participation as well as personal identity and the feeling of continuity all demonstrate close connections to the quality of living conditions (BMFSFJ 1998: 160).

In German research on quality of living conditions in old age a central role is accorded to the maintenance of independence and autonomy (BMFSFJ 1998: 160). Independence could be understood as a result of the interaction between the skills of older people and the specific stimuli and demands of their spatial surroundings. Recent studies show that environmental stimuli and demands both define the spectrum of the skills necessary to be able to lead a life free from help and care and also promote the development of specific skills that contribute to a satisfactory life in old age (Wahl *et al.* 1999; Oswald *et al.* 2000).

In determining quality of living environments, the characteristics of the home and the abilities and skills of older people to lead an autonomous life are interrelated. The objective characteristics of the home usually include: the quality of the sanitary and technical equipment, the structural soundness of the building, barriers within the home, barriers in the immediate surroundings, aids and age-based technology, relative size of the residence, transportation, facilities in the local area (socio-cultural opportunities, shopping opportunities, governmental agencies and social services) as well as support possibilities (Schmitt *et al.* 1994).

There are several methods of recording skills for independent living among older people. As the performance of basal activities (those oriented toward providing basic needs) is essential for independence, the degree of everyday competence is based on daily life activities (ADL) according to Mahoney and Barthel (1965). The analysis of independent living also includes recording instrumental activities (those oriented toward the autonomous management of everyday life). In one study, based on 1092 people aged 60 years and over from the old and new federal states, 23 basal and instrumental activities were recorded (including an exact observation of behaviour during an inspection of the living space, and the performance of individual activities). Several groups of basal and instrumental competencies were found, each of which required different living environments (Kruse and Schmitt 1995; Olbrich 1995).

Furnishing and equipment at home, which maintains or promotes autonomy, is central to but not the sole characteristic of the quality of the living environment. Quality in this respect can also be measured by whether other needs can be satisfied, such as social participation and maintenance of social relationships with members of family, friends and acquaintances, opportunities for privacy, and the protection of personal identity. Many studies point to major divergences between subjectively and objectively assessed quality of living conditions, which can have several causes: adjustment effects, attempts to maintain a positive self-image, processes regulating the level of demands, and the various criteria within objective and subjective perceptions of living conditions. The form of living achieved in old age is the result of the prior history over the lifecourse (BMFSFJ 1998: 160). Satisfaction with one's living space thus depends on personal criteria, desires, preferences and individual history.

Residing in geriatric institutions

Currently 3.8 per cent of older people in Germany aged 75 to 79, 8.2 per cent of those aged 80 to 84, and 17 per cent of those over 90 live in nursing homes, and the majority of them are women (Schneekloth and Müller 2000). The average age of residents in 1998 was 81 and it is rising. The most common reasons for entering a nursing home are: considerably worsening health, collapse of the care situation at home, inability to live independently following a stay in hospital, and the desire not to be a burden on family members (BMFSFJ 2001a). According to Bickel (1995), dementia is the primary health reason for moving to a nursing home. This decision is usually not made freely, and thus the majority of nursing home residents suffer from physical, mental and especially functional health problems. Institutions cannot cure these limitations, but to some extent they can compensate for them so that the illness-based decline in health can be reduced. This compensatory role of institutions for maintaining satisfaction with life has been well documented (Baltes *et al.* 1991; Zank and Baltes 1994,1998).

A particular problem in ensuring subjective QoL in institutions is the adequacy of individual forms of assistance. In addition to the avoidance of specific restrictions of institutional living, age-related needs and their satisfaction must also be considered. Healthy 70 year olds value attractive activities and events in nursing homes differently to 85 year olds who have physical and mental health restrictions. However, 85 per cent of residents are satisfied with institutional life or very satisfied (Wahl and Reichert 1991; Smith *et al.* 1996). The explanation for this discrepancy between objective and subjective reality is that older people, in particular, make use of cognitive adjustment processes that increase their psychological resistance (Staudinger 2000; Staudinger and Greve 2001). This also presents problems in recording QoL in nursing homes.

Predictors of life satisfaction

Closs and Kempe (1986) found five life satisfaction factors among female nursing home residents: social integration versus loneliness, satisfaction with the life situation in old age, subjective physical complaints, calmness versus insecurity or anxiety, and positive life in retrospect. The social integration versus loneliness factor makes it clear that social relationships and activities rank as the most important for satisfaction. Surveys of different scopes for action in nursing homes show, however, that the presence of other people and thus opportunities for social contacts may exist, but they do not automatically contribute to satisfaction with life. Nearly all (98 per cent) nursing home management personnel report that visits are possible throughout the day. However, it was found that only 11 per cent of residents actually received visitors on a daily basis, 36 per cent once or several times per week, 26 per cent one or several times per month, 26 per cent received visitors only infrequently, and 5 per cent received no visitors at all (Schneekloth and Müller 1997). Another study shows that regular visits have a significant positive effect on the wellbeing of nursing home residents with dementia. Improvements were noticed in the mental, physical and social wellbeing of the participants. The visits also eased the suffering resulting from physical illnesses and seemed to reduce the effects that the decline in mental capacities had on residents' capabilities (Oppikofer *et al.* 2002). Numerous intervention studies in nursing homes have attempted to encourage other forms of social activity in addition to visits, including acquiring house pets and organized games (Zank and Baltes 1994).

Autonomy and dependence

The feeling of control and autonomy is essential for dealing successfully with critical life events and for maintaining wellbeing in old age (Baltes 1995; Schwarzer and Knoll 2001). Moving into a nursing home is one such critical life event: giving up one's own home signifies a loss of identity, biographical memories and orientation, and is accompanied by limitations on one's lifestyle. The move is frequently neither foreseeable nor prepared for, so that it can trigger feelings of complete loss of control and depression. There is a significant amount of literature on successful and unsuccessful coping methods in response to this critical life event (Baltes *et al.* 1991).

In response to criticisms of nursing home practice, attempts have been made recently to implement and evaluate interventions. Saup and Schröppel (1993) showed that freedom of choice and opportunities for involvement in environmental changes (for example, arranging living spaces, managing meal times) result in increased wellbeing, satisfaction, and a reduction in hopelessness and emotional irritability. Dependency, a key concept in gerontology, is not a necessary result of ageing but is often created by social and environmental conditions (Baltes 1995). From the perspective of 'learned dependency' (Baltes 1995), observational studies on the interaction between older people and their social partners have shown that behaviour lacking in autonomy resulted in social contacts, whereas autonomous behaviour was ignored at best, if not punished. One goal of this research was to develop a training programme for nursing staff that attempted to achieve behaviour changes in nursing home residents, including changes in attitudes and communication, during contacts between nursing staff and residents (Baltes *et al.* 1994; Zank and Baltes 1994). The results show that there is not only a significant change in the behaviour of trained nursing staff but that training also resulted in the development of autonomous behaviour among the residents.

Interest in quality of living in long-term care facilities was due in part to the introduction of nursing care insurance. Residents' satisfaction and opportunities for independent lifestyles in nursing homes are being used increasingly as criteria for the quality of such homes. One study, for example, highlighted three essential conditions for an independent life in institutions: self-sufficiency, defined as the observance of privacy, dignity, independence, freedom of choice, legal certainty and self-realization; self-determination, which refers to subjective opportunities and the desire to use one's abilities, resources and scope for action. The third criterion is individuality – individual forms of self-reliance and self-determination (Heinemann-Koch *et al.* 1999).

The comprehensive debate following the introduction of nursing care insurance about ensuring quality in nursing homes, leads increasingly to the idea of treating residents as customers. Thus, various customer-oriented instruments are being developed that not only record and evaluate objective QoL in nursing homes but also aim to improve the subjective QoL of older residents. However, the measurement of satisfaction of mentally ill older people, who make up the largest portion of residents, is proving to be a major problem (Aust 1994; BMFSFJ 2001a).

Quality of the neighbourhood

The neighbourhood is a critical element of the living surroundings because it determines the everyday activity radius of older people and thus the extent of their autonomy. Changes in close proximity to the home, for example moving bus or tram stops, closing grocer's shops, or changes in the direction of traffic, can contribute to immobility more quickly than in other phases of life and thus to restrictions in the QoL of older people (Mollenkopf and Flaschenträger 1996).

Participation in social events, opportunities for maintaining existing social relationships and leisure activities or initiating them independently can all be supported by 'senior-friendly environments' (Kruse 1992). Ecological gerontology has found that suitable environments for older people offer not only access to places that provide for their everyday needs, but also enable participation in cultural and social events. Various components of mobility have been studied such as health, agility, availability of a car or access to public transport (Mollenkopf and Flaschenträger 1996). The results make it clear that mobility is the prerequisite for an active and autonomous old age.

As well as offering a resource, the quality of the neighbourhood in old age is also related to other characteristics such as safety outside the home and the availability of informal help. Senior-friendly residential environments can be characterized both by the type and usefulness of structures and by a generation mix that promotes informal support networks. Comparative studies between East and West Germany show that in addition to organizational and environmental qualities such as good medical care and other services, older people also value other characteristics of the neighbourhood, including quiet surroundings, a good environment and transport (Mollenkopf and Flaschenträger 1996).

Technology

New technologies represent one of the most pronounced changes of the last decade in the everyday lives of older people. They can be viewed from the perspective of old age in two ways: their contribution to increasing QoL in old age and their function as a challenge (both positively and negatively) for skills and competencies. The goal of 'technologizing' the everyday life of older people aims at maintaining autonomy. Less attention, however, is given to the negative aspects of technological development, for example where older people lack the skills required to use such devices.

Mollenkopf and Hampel (1994: 25) distinguish several possible contributions of technical innovations to improving QoL in old age:

- Makes some tasks easier as physical strength decreases (for example, household technology).
- Fulfils the need for safety (for example, emergency call systems).
- Compensates for losses in seeing, hearing or motor activity.
- Helps plan leisure time or bridge the gap between periods of being alone.
- Helps initiate and maintain social contacts, even across physical distances.
- Supports one's own caring tasks, or those of third parties, if health is impaired.

There are four perspectives on current research on technology and QoL in old age. First, surveys of the technical equipment in households of older people. The level of care in households of older people with innovations of 'everyday technology' (Münnich and Illgen 1999) and 'gerontological technology' (Mollenkopf 1998) provides information about the acceptance of technology.

Second, the assessment of the usefulness of technical devices for older people such as ticket machines (Rudinger *et al.* 1991; Rudinger 1996). The following main issues exist in terms of the use of technology by older people (Kruse 1992; Mollenkopf and Hampel 1994; Mollenkopf *et al.* 2001):

♦ User-friendliness in operation, handling, functionality (Olbrich 1996).

♦ The problem of 'access' (problems related to information, procurement and financing of technical equipment).

♦ Acceptance (problems of motivation related to using technical innovations; stigmatization of older people through 'age-appropriate' technology).

Evaluation studies using older people as testers of technical equipment have derived specific design guidelines, criteria and user instructions for the construction of new devices (Mollenkopf *et al.* 2001).

Third, the development of new technologies specifically for older people. To enable older people to remain in their own homes as long as possible emphasis has been placed on the development and refinement of intelligent household devices (Meyer and Schulze 1996; Meyer *et al.* 1997). The 'smart house' represents a new technological approach and its special feature is its networking of devices in apartment buildings that were previously isolated (Glatzer *et al.* 1998). Through remote supervision and centralized control of all household appliances new technology contributes to increased safety.

Fourth, studies on the attitudes of older people to technical innovations, such as the acceptance of technology in their own households. One shortcoming in the development of technology for older people consists of its lack of orientation to their lifestyles and values. Many technological innovations are not accepted by older people because they have a 'geriatric' label. Also little consideration is given within product development to the fact that older people belong to different cohorts with different technological competencies.

Health

The term 'health' in old age has two features: health is accorded a high status in old age and the relativity of health becomes a research focus (Kuin *et al.* 2001). Deviating from the biomedical notion of defining health as the absence of disease, good health in old age signifies much more than physical wellbeing. Greater significance is attributed to the subjective state of health; but health also includes dealing adequately with limitations and thereby being able to lead a satisfactory life (Lehr 1997).

German research points to the above average significance of subjective health for QoL in old age and, therefore, objective and subjective states of health are recorded separately. While 'measurable and observable functions as well as the entire spectrum of medical diagnoses are counted' as objective health, subjective health can be summarized as the 'experienced and self-perceived aspects of bodily and mental constitution as well as the subjective judgment of it' (Smith *et al.* 1996: 502). In fact, subjective health is often equated with QoL.[2] Satisfaction with one's own health influences overall life satisfaction, and this in turn is an indication of QoL.

Subjective health and quality of life

The contribution made by health to QoL in later life has been studied extensively (Freund 1995; Freund and Smith 1997; Kuin *et al.* 2001). For 97 per cent of those surveyed between the age of 40 and 85 good health is one of the most important life goals and its importance increases continually during the course of the second half of life (Staudinger *et al.* 1996; Westerhof *et al.* 2001a).

QoL in old age is decisively influenced by subjective health. It also influences how older people manage their own ageing. In a poor state of subjective health, activities (Lehr and Thomae 1987) and social involvement or 'productive activities' decrease (Künemund 2000b). Similarly, the worse one's own state of health is thought to be, the more ageing is experienced as psychophysical loss (Steverink and Timmer 2001).

The Berlin Ageing Study (Mayer and Baltes 1996), the Bonn Gerontological Longitudinal Study (Lehr and Thomae 1987), and the Interdisciplinary Longitudinal Study of the Adult Age (Martin *et al.* 2000) made numerous references to the significance of subjective health for satisfaction, psychophysical wellbeing, and QoL in old age. The Interdisciplinary Longitudinal Study of the Adult Development (ILSE), which began in 1993 in both East and West Germany, emphasizes the great significance both of the global perception of health and the interaction between experienced performance, socio-economic situation and personality characteristics (Rudinger *et al.* 1997; Martin *et al.* 2000; Rietz and Rudinger 2000).

Subjective perceptions of health are also a sensitive indicator of mortality (Lehr and Thomae 1987; Borchelt *et al.* 1996; Smith *et al.* 1996). Even when health-related behaviour and the physical state of health are recorded by medical examinations and laboratory tests, there remains an independent contribution of subjectively perceived health in the prediction of mortality. Some studies have successfully collected data independently on objective and subjective states of health and investigated deviations between the two. Both variables demonstrate significant differences and they reveal different profiles in old age. The results of the Berlin Ageing Study (Mayer and Baltes 1996) show an age-dependent, decreasing significance of the objective state of health for the subjective perception of health. Subjective perceptions remained stable despite an increasingly worse objective state of health during 'ageing in old age' (Borchelt *et al.* 1996).

During the last two decades numerous indices of subjective health-related QoL have been developed (Flick 1998). Their main components include measures for affect and cognitive processes and for physical and social functioning. Current research is concentrating on finding out which criteria older people use to assess their physical and mental health, which subjective theories of health exist, and the way in which self-regulatory approaches contribute to wellbeing (Borchelt *et al.* 1996; Schumacher *et al.* 1997; Fliege and Filipp 2000; Staudinger 2000).

Mental health

Mental health in old age is often linked to healthy and successful ageing and with the development of cognitive status (Baltes *et al.* 1998; Kliegel *et al.* 2001; Martin 2001). According to Helmchen *et al.* (1996) it is not appropriate to speak of mental disorders on a pathological level if, for example, symptoms do not impair everyday functions or subjective wellbeing, because they occur only sporadically or are a short-term reaction to a life event such as bereavement. According to this approach, mental disorders by definition reduce wellbeing and QoL.

Dementia is the most common disorder occurring in the older population and is considered to be one of the most important threats not only to cognitive fitness but to QoL as a whole. The percentage of people over 65 suffering from dementia is 10 per cent to 14 per cent and this increases with age. In the Berlin Ageing Study the prevalence ranged from 2.8 per cent for those 70 to 74 years-of-age to around 35 per cent for those 90 to 94. Among men aged 95 and over there was no further increase and, for women, the risk of dementia increased by a factor of 1.5. This gender-related effect was related to educational level. Dementia was diagnosed more frequently in lower socio-economic groups than in higher ones (Helmchen *et al.* 1996).

The second most frequent form of mental illness in old age is depression; ranging between 9 per cent and 25 per cent. In the Berlin Ageing Study 9 per cent of those aged 70 and over were suffering from depression and there was a significant negative correlation between depressive disorders and subjective wellbeing (Smith *et al.* 1996). The frequency of depression is higher than average among those with mild dementia.

Research on mental health in old age is focused primarily on late old age. For example, the Heidelberg Centenarian Study distinguishes two extreme groups: one that shows no or very minimal loss of cognitive performance and one in which a very strong deficit is evident. The results show that even among very elderly people half remain cognitively intact. The other half of centenarians demonstrate cognitive performance loss, which acts as a significant impediment in everyday life (Kliegel *et al.* 2001; see also Oswald *et al.* 1998; Steinwachs *et al.* 1998).

Mental illnesses have different effects on wellbeing and QoL. Losses in cognitive performance impair the ability of older people to master their everyday life, but there is still little known about specific connections between cognitive disorders and everyday behaviour beyond the routine actions involved in caring for oneself (ADLs). In the Berlin Ageing Study changes were recorded in the everyday behaviour of people with mental illness. The prevalence of overall mental morbidity (DSM-III-R) was relatively high at 24 per cent. In the management of everyday life, daily rhythms and in activities performed, there were clear differences between mentally ill and mentally healthy older people. Indicators of everyday behaviour and competence were recorded in the Yesterday Interview, which reconstructed type, frequency and duration of activities for various aspects of life during the previous day (Moss and Lawton 1982, cited in Helmchen *et al.* 1996).

Leisure time and social activities occupy nearly half (48 per cent) of the time of healthy older people while obligatory activities, such as caring for oneself, running the household and shopping, make up about 38 per cent of the time. On average 28 activities are performed per day that are composed of 13 different activity types. About 80 per cent of these are carried out at home and about 60 per cent are performed alone. Comparing the daily rhythms of mentally ill older people with this average, demented people have significantly more rest periods during the day and spend less time on instrumental activities. The number of different activities performed in everyday life also varies. Demented people have less variety in their activities and spend only half as much time outside the home. Not only is the repertoire of leisure time activities reduced among people with dementia, but also compensation ability is impaired. Discontinued activities are not replaced by others but result in increased rest/sleeping phases during the day. Depressive disorders have hardly any corresponding effects. In their comparison of the role of depression in the QoL among younger and older people, Lang *et al.* (2000) found that depression in older adults (ages 70 to 90) was associated with an increased experience of stress: most older people reported difficulties in managing their everyday lives. Moreover, the wellbeing of older people with depressive illnesses or dementia is impaired due to a comparatively larger number of somatic illnesses, including chronic pain.

Employment and early retirement

Recent studies on the functions and significance of employment in the middle and older adult years begin with the assumption that work represents much more than a source of income. It contributes towards personal identity development, social involvement, and the structuring of everyday life. Schmitt (2001) shows that employed and unemployed people differ both in their subjective experience of the ageing process and across four socio-economic characteristics (subjective state of health, subjectively experienced social integration, net household income and high school diploma). The unemployed experienced their own process of ageing as being influenced strongly by loss of performance levels. They felt less socially integrated and perceived their state of health more pessimistically than the employed.

Satisfaction with work is frequently considered to be an aspect of general satisfaction with life which, in turn, is the cognitive side of wellbeing (Zapf 1984; Zapf 1991). Research, especially in psychology, has concentrated on the negative effects of work such as burdens and demands, rather than on the positive contributions of work to wellbeing. Only since the early 1990s have efforts been made to look at older employees. This research shows that work is not only useful personally (Baltes and Montada 1996) and socially (Künemund 2000a), but will be performed in the future more frequently by older people as a source of income. Policies are proposed aimed at giving older people more opportunities to take part in employment (Naegele and Frerichs 1996) but little research has been conducted on satisfaction with work in old age.

One of the most important methodological problems in measuring work satisfaction is its universally high rating. The increased risk of unemployment with ageing contributes to a situation in which having a job has a misleading influence on the general satisfaction with work. It must be assumed that there are a large number of those who are 'satisfied but resigned' (Zapf 1991). Resigned satisfaction, however, can hardly be accepted as an indicator of subjective wellbeing (Frese 1990).

Entering retirement

The significance of work in a person's biography and its contribution to increasing QoL must be reevaluated as older people move beyond employment. Early departure from working life lessens the opportunities to participate in society and raises the question whether this should be compensated by other forms of involvement (Kohli *et al.* 1993; Niederfranke 1996; Kohli and Künemund 1997, 2000). Recent studies on wellbeing after entering retirement show that most older people are able to replace lost social relationships in employment with other social contacts (Mayring 2000). However, subjective evaluations of retirement depend on societal attitudes to retirement (Westerhof 2001a).

Recent research has concentrated on changes in the life situation associated with the termination of employment (Lehr and Niederfranke 1991; Naegele 1992; Mayring 2000). There are no important changes in health. Retirement does have an impact on income, social relationships, and the reorganization of everyday life. On average income falls by 25 to 30 per cent (Maier 2000). Social relationships and contacts must be redesigned. In retirement available contacts and interests are strengthened; there is seldom an engagement in completely new activities. Although the life situation changes after entering retirement, such changes do not lead to a reduction in wellbeing among those affected (Mayring 2000). The following are the essential factors that influence wellbeing in retirement:

◆ The *anticipation of entering retirement*, a positive attitude about life without work, as well as concrete plans for organizing this phase of life (Saup and Mayring 1995).

◆ *Characteristics of the previous work situation.* A high degree of satisfaction with previous employment relieves reorientation retirement. A similarly high degree of wellbeing was shown by people who have reached their private goals (for example, family life) and find instrumental and emotional support in their social relationships (Abraham 1993; Mayring 2000).

◆ *The type of transition to retirement.* The transition to early retirement is more likely to be free of conflicts where employers' policies are oriented toward consensus and the interests of older employees (Teipen and Zierep 1996). The end of professional life is perceived as being more negative the earlier, more involuntarily and sudden the change is made.

◆ *Wellbeing before retirement.* This is connected with several personality variables such as optimism, emotional stability and a positive view of old age (Westerhof 2001b) and is a predictor of subjective wellbeing *after* retirement (Mayring 2000).

The main finding of many recent studies is that entering retirement does not necessitate an overall decline in the state of health. Satisfaction with life, happiness and freedom from burdens remains constant both prior to and after entering retirement. Behind the relatively constant picture of satisfaction with life, however, differences exist between particular domains. Thus entering retirement means gains in leisure time, but also losses in societal status, financially and in network satisfaction (Mayring 2000).

Socio-economic status

In addition to health, socio-economic status, measured by income, assets and educational level, is one of the main determinants of QoL in old age. Research based on the Welfare Survey (WS) and the Socio-Economic Panel (SOEP) has demonstrated links between material resources and subjective wellbeing. It is much more difficult to record individuals' assets than income because there are no reliable data (Fachinger 1998; Motel 2000). However, national data point to the increasing significance of assets in old age and to differences in the distribution of assets (Naegele 2000; Fachinger 1998, 2001).

Many surveys show that good living conditions lead to a higher degree of subjective wellbeing (Glatzer and Volkert 1980; Zapf 1994; Delhey and Böhnke 1999). The occurrence of multiple problems leads to lower satisfaction with life in old age (Mathwig and Mollenkopf 1996). Sociological research also points to the significance of material resources for QoL in old age (Naegele 1998). Social gerontology treats income and health as the essential determining factors for participation in social events, integration, and autonomy in old age (Naegele 1998).

Material factors, such as income, are also of central significance for psychological health and perceived QoL in old age. Whether ageing is experienced as a phase of 'late freedom' or as its opposite, is associated significantly with the social status of older people (Schmitt 2000, quoted in Pohlmann 2001: 76). Low income and loneliness, in particular, lead to old age being experienced as a psychophysical breakdown. Educational level, in contrast, contributes both to the development of a 'younger' age identity and, especially, to whether ageing is interpreted as a matter of personal growth (Steverink and Timmer 2001).

Epidemiological research shows that a higher mortality rate is evidence of increasing inequalities in living conditions (Walter and Schwartz 2001). The

SOEP, for example, records class-specific differences in mortality rates and life expectancy and also studies survival curves based on age, gender and income (Voges 1996, in Walter and Schwartz 2001: 163). Theories of self-efficacy[3] are used as explanations for the differences in life expectancy as determined by socio-economic status. Other explanations are related to the availability of public support. Social activities seem to reduce the mortality risk (Steinbach 1992, quoted by Walter and Schwartz 2001: 163).

Inequalities in quality of life

Socio-economic status

Regional variations in socio-economic status in Germany exist due to the as yet incomplete process of unification. Existing disparities in terms of income and assets are reflected in the perceived QoL and satisfaction with life of those affected (Schwitzer 1995; Hauser *et al.* 1996; Mathwig and Mollenkopf 1996; Delhey and Böhnke 1999). Older people in East Germany are not affected in the same way by the unequal distribution of income. While early retirees who were affected by long-term unemployment, but also some of those advanced in years, are disadvantaged in terms of their income, retired persons and pensioners who have especially long contribution years are seen as 'winners of the system' (Hauser *et al.* 1996: 306). Although their income was significantly above average in comparison with other income groups in East Germany, they are also disadvantaged relative to West Germans (for example, they were not able to acquire assets).

Differences in income exist not only between the old and new federal states but also between the genders. Lower pensions are found among women, especially very elderly women and those living alone (Naegele 1998; Fachinger 2001). The inequality between women and men in terms of old-age income is even more pronounced in the West than in the East. This reflects the different periods of insurance of those affected (Fachinger 2001).

Another group of people affected by a low level of material comfort is foreign immigrants. Differences exist in relationship to ethnic identity, date of immigration or the respective legal status. Different legal statuses also mean different options for participating in the job market. German immigrants from Eastern Europe are in a privileged position compared to other immigrant groups. They are considered equal to the local populations legally and politically, and also in terms of access to the job market, and thus are not a particularly disadvantaged group even in old age (Seifert 1996). The date of immigration also plays a role in terms of income, so that the immigrants themselves must be subdivided into different cohorts. For example, the group of older foreign immigrants of the first guestworker generation who today are in their third age, were subject to specific risks, for example, a high rate of unemployment, which continue to have an effect today (Seifert 1996). Nothing can be said about the subjective QoL of older immigrants. In most of the representative surveys, with the exception of the SOEP, this group is not recorded and other research has only recently been initiated.

Health

Women tend to assess their health more negatively than men. A key factor here is their higher life expectancy and thus more frequent encounter with mobility limitations and comorbidity. There are no systematic comparative studies of the health-related QoL of older immigrants. What evidence there is suggests that the state of health of this group is generally poor. Various reasons are given for this: low income and low levels of formal education, greater impact on unemployment and accumulation of health-related burdens over the course of working life, poor living conditions, and the stress triggered by immigration (Dietzel-Papakyriakou 1998).

Quality of living conditions

Good residential environments are unequally distributed regionally. Disparities exist between East and West Germany and between urban and rural areas (Scheewe 1996). In East Germany older people suffer from poor living conditions, for example, lack of sanitary facilities, deficiencies in the structural soundness of the buildings, and relatively high rents (Hauser et al. 1996; Hinrichs 1997, 1999). The access of older people to the surrounding resources in rural areas, especially in the Eastern states, continues to be poor (Motel et al. 2000). Mollenkopf and Flaschenträger (1996) show that feelings of insecurity in the neighbourhood are especially pronounced at night, and especially among women. Feelings of poor security occur among people in the downtown areas of cities much more frequently than for those in the outskirts.

Among older women poor living conditions occur more frequently alongside other deficiencies in the living situation such as lower income, poor health and social isolation. This is especially true of women who are very elderly and live alone (Mathwig and Mollenkopf 1996). The living situation of older immigrants is different from that of the older German population. Older ethnic minority groups are less likely to own their residences, they live in homes that are less well equipped, and their living space is smaller. High rents and the structural supply shortage of their neighbourhoods further diminish the quality of living conditions (BMFSFJ 1998).

Social relationships

East-West comparisons show that older people in East Germany are more satisfied with their family relationships than older people in the West (Hauser *et al.* 1996). This is attributed to differences in socialization and the resulting deviation of meaning in family networks. In the former GDR the family served the individual as the only source of privacy, as a niche outside the reach of governmental control. This is reflected in the closeness experienced by different generations. Thus, East German parents report especially close and satisfying relationships with their children (Szydlik 2000). These findings do not, however, allow conclusions to be drawn about the specific needs of older people in the East or West, or about the practical role played by the family in East Germany.

More older people in East Germany report feelings of loneliness than is the case for those in West Germany. This is particularly true for women. East Germans report a lack of contact with people of the same age. Relationships with fellow employees could not be maintained following retirement. This lack of social integration is also reflected in the social contact behaviour of older people in East Germany. Compared with West Germans, East Germans more frequently do without activities outside the home (Schröder 1995) and therefore without opportunities to make new contacts.

Among older women an exclusively family-centred lifestyle contributes more to dissatisfaction than to satisfaction (Lehr and Minnemann 1987). Married women are especially dissatisfied with their lives if they say that marriage and family is their sole purpose in life (Everwien 1992). Single women more frequently mention contacts outside the family as essential factors for their satisfaction with life and prove generally to be more satisfied.

The negative correlation between the size of older women's network and their happiness (Niederfranke 1991) is explained by the fact that women not only receive more social support in social relationships but also provide more support (Saup 1991), some of which is burdensome. The Berlin Ageing Study (Mayer and Baltes 1996), in contrast, finds no differences in social integration between men and women among the very elderly in terms of the size and structure of the social network as well as the link between network size, social support and subjective wellbeing. Women have higher values than men just for experienced loneliness but this is explained by marital status and living situation and not by sex (Baltes *et al.* 1996a).

Only descriptive data exist on the social networks of older ethnic minority groups. They point to an orientation towards important relationships in the same ethnic group, which increase in old age (Dietzel-Papakyriakou and Olbermann 1996). Whether this strategy corresponds to the needs of older immigrants themselves, or whether it is a result of failed integration and exclusion, cannot be determined. Several studies point to an increase in the effectiveness of culture-specific norms in old age. Thus, children of older immigrants report a special closeness to, and responsibility for, their own older parents (Szydlik 2000).

Quality of living after retirement

Transitions to retirement have become very heterogeneous. Variations can be seen, for example, at the time the occupation is terminated as well as with the modes of transition upon entering retirement. There are specific patterns for the transition to retirement that are dependent upon gender and region.

Older employees in the East are much more threatened or affected by the risk of unemployment and re-employment is rare after the age of 55. Lower incomes likewise have a negative effect on the QoL of older early retirees, and this is reflected in other indicators of QoL such as home furnishings or owner-ship of consumer durables (Hauser *et al.* 1996). The most dissatisfied are those people who previously had a relatively high household income (Hauser *et al.* 1996). Unemployment and early retirement represent new and undesirable experiences for the population in the Eastern states. While early retirees in the Western states increasingly mention the positive sides of the postwork phase of life, their Eastern counterparts belong to the reconstruction generation of the former GDR whose typical biography was strongly oriented to work. As the transition to retirement was not voluntary it is generally assessed as being negative. Contacts outside the family with people of the same age are found wanting, and feelings of social marginalization and uselessness increase. New life goals are sought especially in the family but cannot be realized satis-factorily due to a reorientation of younger generations (Genz 1995). The transition to early retirement in the new states is heavily burdened with conflict for the majority of older people (Ernst 1996). They report a lack of control over this process. Initially, income was the chief cause of concern but later the emphasis was shifted to deficits of a social nature (Hauser *et al.* 1996).

The point at which women leave employment is often determined by their partners or families. With the adjustment to female retirement, forms of social inequality that result from the middle phase of life, become longer and stronger (Clemens 1995). Gender-specific inequalities in income and in career organization (Naegele 1992) are reflected in standard of living as well as perceived QoL.

The post-occupational phase of life has become gender-specific – the 'female retirement'. As Clemens (1995) shows, the family and professional biography, health-related and financial prerequisites influence the quality of adjustment to retirement. Women, especially those who are single or divorced, have to deal with particularly serious limitations to their income (Maier 2000). This is also reflected in the subjective wellbeing and the satisfaction with life of older women (Hauser *et al.* 1996; Mayring 2000). Married women have more favourable prospects than single or divorced women, or those living separately, in terms of making adjustments to life after retirement.

Conclusion

In Germany, research on quality of life in in old age is based on different trad-itions: socio-economic research, research into psychological and health-oriented wellbeing, and gerontological research on the concept of successful ageing. The resulting different theoretical diversity regarding QoL and the different conceptualizations of QoL in old age have stimulated a great deal of empirical research but have led to outcomes that cannot be compared with each other. The consequences are a considerable number of research studies addressing different dimensions of a good life in old age as well as an increasing number of theoretical questions that can be viewed as unresolved. One of them concerns the definition of individual dimensions of a good life as well as their relative weighting with increasing age. In particular, there is a need for further empirical research about subjective criteria of quality of life from the perspective of older persons.

Notes

1. The Welfare Survey (WS) and the Socio-Economic Panel (SOEP) are representative surveys for measuring welfare and recording QoL with their objective and subjective components (Habich *et al.* 1999: 2). The Welfare Survey has been conducted at regular intervals since 1978 (in East Germany since 1990; the last recording took place in 1998) and is among the most important instruments for observing societal dynamics over the long term. The Socio-economic Panel is a repeat survey that has been conducted annually since 1984; it currently includes 7000 households. The German Ageing Survey is a repeated interdisciplinary survey of 5000 men and women aged 40–85.

2. The World Health Organization creates an exemplary connection between health and wellbeing (subjective QoL) by defining health as a 'state of complete physical, mental and social wellbeing' (WHO 1947, quoted by Smith *et al.* 1996: 502). This wording, however, conveys the fact that it is less of an empirical factor and more normative, 'a good that people strive for but actually never achieve' (Kickbusch 1999: 275).

3. Self-efficacy refers to the assessment of an individual in terms of his or her ability to successfully carry out a specific behaviour (Bandura 1992, quoted by Walter and Schwartz 2001: 163). A high degree of self-efficacy is associated with increased preventative behaviour and a positive assessment of one's own health.

3

Italy: quality of life in old age I

Francesca Polverini and Giovanni Lamura

Introduction

Italy is currently regarded as one of the oldest countries in the world (Kinsella and Velkoff 2001), with the over 65 year olds comprising 18.6 per cent of the population (ISTAT 2003: 32), but debate on the issue of quality of life (QoL) in older age has seldom been approached in a systematic way. In recent years research has been devoted to the study of ageing and QoL from different points of view: psychological, medical, economic and financial. Multidisciplinary studies are rare, so pinpointing the key factors promoting quality in later life is a complex task.

Definition and measurement of quality of life

The concept of wellbeing, often used as a synonym for QoL, has in the past been strongly linked to income or, more generally, to the presence of adequate means (material, relational, psychophysical, environmental). Only recently has greater importance been attributed to wellbeing as the quality of receiving satisfaction from the use of available resources, and not only from their mere possession, an approach that emphasizes the importance of individual lifestyle and personal choice (Sen 1993).

Despite this positive development, the general approach underlying most national studies conducted on this topic in Italy is still based on economic considerations (Frey 1999, 2002). Not surprisingly, therefore, the most common definitions of QoL in Italy use average per capita income (Livraghi 1997) and, specifically, the relative poverty threshold for a family of two people (about 823 euros a month in 2002).

The most popular approach among Italian scholars is the medical-psychological one, according to which the concept of QoL in old age is dominated by health. Here the evaluation of wellbeing during the last phase of life takes place on the basis of an individual's psychophysical conditions, with particular regard to disease, disability and mental functioning. The use of assessment criteria that, in practice, link the QoL to the older person's functional-cognitive-psychological capacity and compare it to the levels recorded in the adult population has probably contributed to the spread of a negative perception of old age by emphasizing a close correlation between physical and cognitive performances and QoL.

The strictly medical approach (functional-cognitive) was common in the past and the psychological approach has become more popular over the last three decades (Cesa-Bianchi and Cristini 1998). In Italy the latter approach has fostered an interpretative model of QoL that integrates objective and subjective factors, starting from the assumption that the overall level of wellbeing is strongly influenced by how objective living conditions are perceived by the individual, and by the degree of satisfaction derived from them. Although some comprehensive examples of this approach have been developed recently (Regione Veneto 2002), their application has usually been limited to local areas, therefore providing little insight on the overall situation in Italy, a country that is notoriously characterized by deep territorial differences.

Some recent examples of application at the national level of this more integrated approach to QoL, attempting to take into account different kinds of indicators, are those of Laicardi and colleagues (1987, 2000) and of Vitali (2002, 2003), as well as by the leading Italian economic newspaper, *Il Sole – 24 Ore* (2003). Laicardi identified the following four basic factors of wellbeing for people in older age:

- *material factors*: income availability and opportunity to take advantage of certain services;

- *environmental factors*: characteristics of the home and neighbourhood (access to services, degree of security and criminality), mental approach and ability to avail oneself of new technologies; political and social assets;

- *relational factors*: family, friends and social networks, social, political and religious integration, free time, social role after retirement and previous working activity;

- *individual factors*: psychophysical health condition, and subjective perception of one's own situation.

Although these factors were identified as early as the mid 1980s, their integration and practical use for data collection purposes has remained limited. In contrast, the approach followed more recently by some major Italian economic journals – such as *Il Sole – 24 Ore* and *Italia Oggi* – focuses on a complex set of theoretical assumptions that have been operationalized in statistical terms, providing the basis for periodical surveys on QoL in Italy (Vitali 2002 and 2003, *Il Sole – 24 Ore* 2003). These annual surveys monitoring territorial differences, in areas such as work and business, environment, criminality, population, services, leisure time, life standards, personal feelings, are used to build a QoL rating for all 103 Italian provinces.

Although these surveys have been able to provide interesting information on spatial differences in QoL, their reliance on available statistics, such as unemployment rates, suicide rates or availability of hospital beds, remains a major limitation. Furthermore, so far they have not provided any information regarding the QoL of subgroups of populations such as older people. Even worse, they use some indicators, such as death rates, as synonyms for low QoL, thus implicitly giving a negative weight to a higher percentage of older people within the total population.

A more recent and innovative approach, for Italy at least, has been provided by the European Study on Adult Wellbeing (ESAW), a research project funded by the European Commission, aimed at identifying which of the following factors, along with personal characteristics and culture, exert a direct causal contribution to the outcome variable *ageing well*: physical health and functional status; self resources; life activity; material security; and social support. The project, which is part of a wider Global Ageing Initiative initiated by the Indiana University Center on Aging and Aged (USA), was carried out in 2002 and 2003 in six European countries (Austria, Italy, Luxembourg, The Netherlands, Sweden and the UK), where representative national samples of 1800 to 2000 over 50 year olds enabled the building of a European sociocultural model (Ferring *et al.* 2003a). This was accomplished through the use of selected indicators, covering each of the five domains, to predict how variation in life satisfaction is explained by the chosen components. The comparative findings deriving from the ESAW study, presented later, show that such an approach can identify which factors play a major role in influencing wellbeing levels in a society, in subgroups of the population and even in cross-national samples (Scharf *et al.* 2003).

Finally, a major fault of most sources of data concerning QoL in Italy is the tendency to consider the older population as one broad category, rather than dividing it into different age groups. Most Italian data cover only people over 65, while others, at best, disaggregate information into two age groups: 65 to 75 and over 75. This represents an obstacle to any attempt at in-depth analysis of the changes occurring in the perception of wellbeing among older people.

Environments of ageing

For many older Italians ageing is associated with a reduction in the use of both spatial and relational environments, so that the home and the neighbourhood, family and friends become more significant for them (Lazzarini 1994). The home, in particular, represents for the current generation of older Italians, a powerful symbol of local belonging. The fact that they tend to spend more time indoors, especially in the case of older women, intensifies the affective tie with their own home and the desire to make it as safe and comfortable as possible. This explains the high importance of the home and residential setting to older Italians' QoL.

As for housing, many factors considered unimportant in younger age, such as the presence (or lack) of a lift in the building, can become essential with ageing. Empirical evidence shows, however, that the housing conditions of older Italians are on average worse than for the general population. A survey by SPI-CGIL (1997) points out that the risk of housing deprivation mainly concerns people over 75, an age group also characterized in most cases by low income, restrictions on personal autonomy and a high probability of living alone. Other studies confirm that older people's houses tend to be substandard and less safe, often presenting architectural barriers with old-fashioned interior design. A national survey carried out by the Italian Forum of Municipal Social Services (1997) found that over two-thirds (68 per cent) of older people's households had no lift and about a quarter (24 per cent) had no effective heating system, whereas 2 per cent still had outdoor lavatories. A subsequent survey showed that 40 per cent of people over 65 lived on the upper floors of buildings with no lift, and many older people experienced difficulties in performing the activities of daily living such as climbing stairs (45 per cent), going out (27 per cent) and carrying heavy objects (32 per cent) (Marcellini *et al.* 1999: 73).

Almost all older Italians (98 per cent) live in private houses (Lamura *et al.* 2003: 27). Since older people have a lower than average income, it is easy to understand that many of them cannot face the heavy expenses entailed in the restoration of their homes (ISTAT 2001a). This increases the risk for older people of exposure to domestic accidents: in 1999 those over 65 made up 26 per cent of the 3,048,000 victims of such accidents (ISTAT 1999a), and 76 per cent of casualties due to domestic accidents (and older people only make up 18 per cent of the whole population). These data reflect the gravity of a situation that implies huge economic and social costs, amounting to an annual expenditure of at least 670 million euros for the National Health Service simply for admissions to hospitals due to fractures caused by domestic accidents (ISTAT 2000c). Falls are the main cause of accidents among older people (43.7 per cent against 28.8 per cent in the whole population), who comprise almost all of those (96.7 per cent) who die as the consequence of a fall.

Recently some significant initiatives have been taken, including a policy of tax allowances for the restoration of buildings, in order to prevent domestic accidents and guarantee greater security against a third party, the institution of housewives' compulsory insurance against domestic accidents, and the launch of several advertising campaigns about safety in the home aimed at older people (Chapter 8). Despite these and other recent initiatives, the lack of security of older people at home remains one of the main barriers to the improvement of QoL in Italy.

Although the topic of safe housing was not included in the items analysed by the ESAW study, other dimensions related to housing are relevant to QoL (Lamura *et al.* 2003: 26ff). One of these concerns the role of house ownership for life satisfaction, confirming that owning one's own home is strongly correlated to higher levels of wellbeing, thus positively impacting on older Italians' QoL. Older Italians are among those with the highest percentages of home ownership in Europe and the lowest levels of mortgages still to be paid. According to this study, older Italians are also underrepresented among those who live in public housing or receive a rent subsidy – a condition that is cross-nationally a strong predictor of lower life satisfaction – which emphasizes the marginal role played by housing policies in Italy.

Residential and nursing homes

Like other Mediterranean countries the proportion of Italian older people living in residential settings (nursing homes and older people's homes) is much lower than in Central and Northern Europe (Nimwegen and Moors 1997; Tomassini *et al.* 2004). According to census data, this figure was 1.9 per cent of the over 65-year-old population in 1981 and 1.6 per cent in 1991, and at present it is estimated to be not much higher or even decreasing, with even lower percentages in the southern regions of Italy (Pace 1996; Tomassini *et al.* 2004).

These data are explained by the still relatively consistent family network, associated with a system of values that makes the nursing or older people's home a last resort both in relatives' and older people's eyes. For example, a recent survey of family caregivers found that 87 per cent are against this solution, and only in a real case of necessity (4 per cent of all cases) would they consider it (Mengani *et al.* 1999: 108). Older people generally have great expectations of help from their children and one of their main fears is ending up in a nursing home (Ministero dell Interno 1994). The low demand/supply of residential and nursing homes in Italy is further explained by the increase in the number of older people being cared for in their own homes by foreign immigrants, of whom in the last decade several hundreds of thousands have been hired (Caritas and Migrantes 2003; Socci *et al.* 2003). This development, which allows the older person to keep on living in his/her own home (Golini and Calvani 1997), is also a relatively cheap one, since the salary of a foreign care worker cohabiting with the older person rarely exceeds 800–1000 euros per month, compared to the 1200–1500 euros per month for a nursing home. The main reasons why older people resort to a residential home is a reduction in their autonomy coupled with the decreasing support capacities of Italian families. This explains why, though many Italian residential homes are not adequately equipped, the presence of older disabled people is very high, while self-sufficient people or slightly disabled people only account for 2.6 per cent and 29.8 per cent of the total, against 34.1 per cent and 47 per cent of people living in their own homes (Renzi *et al.* 1995).

As far as the relationship between QoL and residential settings is concerned, studies conducted on older patients in long-term care institutions have shown that there exists a positive correlation between being able to keep frequent contacts with and to rely on the support of a family network and the psychosocial condition of institutionalized older people, as this makes them more willing to accept the fact of living there (Ranieri *et al.* 2000). Therefore, among the factors for the assessment of older people's QoL in residential institutions, a central role is played by human relations in general, and by the relationships with the staff of the nursing home in particular (Franci and Corsi 1996).

An extremely relevant factor for QoL in older age in general, and especially for those in nursing homes, is the ability to maintain an optimum level of physical activity. Despite the evidence of the effectiveness of such activity, which demonstrates how after long periods of physical inactivity there still persists the ability to respond to functional stimuli and that many very elderly people are still keen on physical activities (Schena, Martinelli and Noro 2000), its practice in nursing homes is rare (Paciaroni 2000: 66).

It is also important in nursing homes to maintain psychological wellbeing. Experimental studies conducted in residential homes have pointed to the effectiveness of psychosocial, rehabilitative, speech therapy, physiotherapy and recreational practices, as opposed to pharmacological interventions in the care of older people affected by depression (Ferilli *et al.* 2000). Research has shown not only that the use of anti-depression drugs is associated with the risk of thighbone fractures (Sgadari *et al.* 2000), but also that older people living in institutions are generally more depressed than those who live in their own homes, even when the living conditions in the residential settings appear to be fully satisfactory in the eyes of outsiders (Cataldi 1996). Thus the Italian NHS for several years has had among its aims the prevention of accidents among old inpatients in nursing homes, including a reduction in the number and quantity of drugs administered (Allegato al Piano Sanitario Nazionale 1998–2000).

A real contribution to the improvement in older people's QoL in residential settings could be achieved by helping them to maintain their personal autonomy by the personalization of rooms, for instance allowing them to furnish their rooms with personal furniture and goods, giving them the opportunity to go out and receive friends, to cook their meals and the maintenance of contacts with their families and the outside world in general (Franci and Corsi 1996: 58).[1] Also it would be advisable to open nursing homes to the local community by making internal services available to outsiders, such as volunteers' meeting points, social and recreational centres for the older people of the area, soft gym programmes, information centres and any other initiative that may put older inpatients and young people in touch, for instance by offering students' accommodation in nursing homes, or setting up cafeterias open to the general public (SPI-CGIL 1990: 215).

Turning to the technologies linked to nursing homes, four elements seem to be of primary importance for the QoL of disabled older people (Monzeglio 1996):

◆ spaces and their functions must be *easily recognizable*: clear instructions must be given to allow inpatients to move around easily inside the nursing home and to identify different areas and functions, avoiding the anonymous features of formal care structures;

◆ spaces must be *easily accessible*: both with reference to the nursing home as a whole and to the different areas and rooms;

- the nursing home should be *flexible*: any inpatient should be able to enjoy it, thanks to the adaptability of both furniture and space use to their different needs;

- the nursing home should be *secure*: there should not be any dangerous steps or passages; doors and locks should be operated without any difficulty; doors should be made easily recognizable; lifts and stairs should be clearly indicated; there should be rounded off corners and uninterrupted banisters.

Despite substantial progress in environmental psychology – for example, in identifying the importance of colours to improve the possibility of recognizing places in case of sight impairment, or in combining comfort and pleasantness of rooms and spaces with security – currently very few older people's homes apply such evidence in practice.

Quality of neighbourhood

Security and crime

A major element in the quality of their neighbourhood is older people's perception of the security it offers them. Research by the Italian National Statistical Institute (ISTAT), reported in Tables 3.1, 3.2 and 3.3, shows the following.

In the streets (Table 3.1, cols 2–3): women feel insecure when walking alone in the dark, and therefore feel forced to take precautions at twice the rate of men. The proportion feeling insecure and taking precautions tends to increase with age, peaking in the age group 55–64 (the decrease among those over 65 is to be seen in the light of the decline in the number of those who go out regularly).

At home (Table 3.1, cols 3–6): the percentage of people who feel insecure at home is lower than in the streets and, again, women feel less secure than men (col. 3). The proportion of those who do not feel secure and shut themselves up in the house or regularly check whether there are any intruders, is higher among the over 65s because they are more sedentary and thus more sensitive to threats indoors (cols 3–5).

Although the feeling of insecurity due to the perception of criminal episodes in the neighbourhood very seldom results in moving to a different area, especially among people aged over 65 (Table 3.2, col. 1–2), a high number of people experience feelings of being neglected by the police (col. 6), and complain about the lack of law enforcement in the neighbourhood.

Bag snatching and pickpocketing are reported less frequently among older people (Table 3.3, col. 1–3). The percentage of men who report bag snatching (col. 2) is in fact low among people under 44 years of age, and rises in

Table 3.1 Perception of security and precautions taken at night in the street or at home by those over 35 years, 1997–98 (per 100 persons of same age and sex)

	1 Feels very or totally insecure when walking alone at dark (a).		2 Takes precautions when walking in the dark and avoids people and certain streets (b).		3 Feels very or totally insecure when alone at home at dark (c).		4 Often or always locks the door if alone at home during the day (d).		5 Often or always checks if there are any intruders when coming back home (d).		6 Often or always checks if there are any intruders on hearing noises in the house (d).	
Age group	M	F	M	F	M	F	M	F	M	F	M	F
35–44	14.3	38.1	26.5	51.2	4.6	12.4	29.7	42.3	14.0	17.9	50.6	54.3
45–54	17.2	39.3	29.5	47.8	4.2	15.1	28.7	44.7	13.9	19.1	49.6	53.5
55–64	21.8	42.3	31.8	46.7	6.3	20.3	34.4	52.7	18.2	22.0	51.1	51.3
65 and over	24.5	36.7	29.8	34.5	9.5	21.8	46.6	65.7	20.5	24.3	47.7	45.7
Total (e)	17.3	39.6	29.4	49.2	5.5	17.6	31.4	49.5	16.2	22.3	51.6	54.3

Notes:

a) possible answers: very, quite, little, not at all, never goes out

b) possible answers: no, yes, don't know, don't remember, never goes out

c) possible answers: very, quite, little, not at all

d) possible answers: never, seldom, often, always

e) per 100 people of same sex and older than 14

Source: ISTAT (1999a).

Table 3.2 Perception of criminal events in the neighbourhood by population aged 35 and over, 1997–98 (per 100 persons of same age and sex)

Age group	1 Moved to a different house for fear of criminal events.		2 Is going to move to a different house for fear of criminal events.		3 Defines his/her neighbourhood very or quite insecure (a).		4 Often sees drug addicts taking drugs(b).		5 Is often witness to acts of vandalism against public property (b).		6 The police seldom or never patrol the neighbourhood (a).	
	M	F	M	F	M	F	M	F	M	F	M	F
35–44	1.5	1.6	3.0	3.4	23.4	24.7	8.2	7.1	14.7	14.0	40.9	46.4
45–54	1.4	1.8	2.1	2.7	22.8	22.6	9.1	6.9	12.9	12.1	41.4	45.8
55–64	0.9	0.9	1.6	2.2	22.4	22.6	10.8	7.3	15.9	11.4	42.0	43.9
65 and over	0.5	0.8	1.1	1.2	19.5	21.7	6.5	5.1	9.9	8.0	36.1	36.6
Total (c)	**1.1**	**1.3**	**2.1**	**2.5**	**22.7**	**23.7**	**8.9**	**6.9**	**14.1**	**12.8**	**40.2**	**44.0**

Notes:

Possible answers:

a) very, quite, little, not at all

b) often, sometimes, seldom, never

c) 100 people of the same sex and aged over 14

Source: ISTAT (1999a).

Table 3.3 People over 35 years pickpocketed or bagsnatched in the last 12 months, 2000 (%)

Age group	1 Victims of bag snatching (a).		2 Reported cases of bag snatching (b).		3 Victims of pick pocketing (a).		4 Reported cases of pick pocketing (b).		5 Persons perceiving an increase in criminality level (c).	
	M	F	M	F	M	F	M	F	M	F
35–44	0.8	1.0	38.4	64.8	1.7	2.1	55.4	67.6	15.5	15.3
45–54	0.8	1.4	51.4	57.5	1.7	1.8	58.1	66.7	16.1	16.0
55–64	0.9	2.0	58.7	64.7	1.2	2.8	59.8	54.1	17.6	17.1
65 and over	0.4	1.3	64.7	64.0	1.2	1.6	57.5	45.4	14.1	13.7
Total (d)	**0.8**	**1.3**	**54.3**	**61.0**	**1.6**	**2.1**	**56.0**	**58.1**	**15.4**	**15.1**

Notes:
a) per 100 people
b) per 100 people victims of bag snatching or pick pocketing with reference to the last episode reported to the police
c) possible answers: increase, the same, decrease, I never go out
d) per 100 people of the same sex and older than 14.
Source: ISTAT (2000a).

the older age groups, while remaining high among women; in the case of pickpocketing, the trend is completely different: the proportion of women who report this crime decreases as they grow older, while that of men remains constant on a medium-high percentage. The reasons for this trend are not clear and it requires further research. The fact that women over 65 tend to give up reporting cases of pickpocketing is remarkable because the over 65 population is generally more firmly against criminality and asks for 'more severe penalties and punishments' (55 per cent) more frequently than do people aged between 35 and 44 (CNEL 2000: 30).

The findings emerging from the ESAW study provide a comparative confirmation of the relatively lower sense of security felt by many older Italians, who are the highest percentage of respondents (6.2 per cent) who 'do not feel safe in the place where they live' (Lamura et al. 2003: 28). This is important because this sense of (in)security is strongly correlated to overall life satisfaction (Lamura et al. 2003: 42), thus emphasizing that policy intervention in this field is urgently needed in Italy.

Accessibility to services

The quality of a neighbourhood also depends on the availability and accessibility of services. The ISTAT has studied the usage by the population of four main services: the Registry Office, the Azienda Sanitaria Locale (ASL, that is the local offices of the NHS), the post office and the bank. The data only show how many people actually went to these offices over the last 12 months and not the overall use, such as via a third party, therefore a low percentage here might reflect mobility problems rather than need.

The service most attended by older people is the post office, followed by the bank for men in the age group 65–74, and by the ASL for men aged over 75 and for women of all age groups. The centrality of the post office is due to the fact that in Italy pensions are traditionally cashed at post offices, thus a decrease in the use of this service is registered only among people over 75. There is a marked decline in the use of a bank among people in their early sixties. Banks are generally attended by a higher percentage of men than women in any age range, but the attendance undergoes a steady decline on the part of women in the age group 60–4 (49 per cent 60–4; 40.4 per cent 65–74; 25.7 per cent 75 and over compared with 55.1 per cent 55–9), and on the part of men over 65 (67 per cent 65–74; 47.1 per cent 75 and over compared with 79.2 per cent 55–9).

Out of the four services studied, the ASL is the least used by men aged 55–9 and the second least used by women (after the Registry Office), but it becomes the most attended by people over 75 after the post office. This is because of a real increase in the use of this service on the part of men, and of a less steady decline on the part of women (limited to women over 75) than in the use of the other three services. The location of these services can become crucial for older people's QoL and their closure in small centres or in areas considered to be of lesser importance would have a different impact on subgroups of older people.

Transport

Transport does not seem to affect the QoL of Italian older people very significantly. This does not mean, however, that it is unimportant. The most common form of public transport used by older people is the coach (used by 87 per cent), followed by the bus or tram (63 per cent), the train (60 per cent) and the underground (10 per cent), while the car (58 per cent) is the most common private means of transport (SPI-CGIL/CER 1997: 75). As for the favourite means of transport, the majority in the age range 60–74 prefer public transport (29 per cent), while people over 75 prefer the 'on foot' option (24 per cent). In the latter age group 13 per cent of people are usually accompanied when going out, against an average of 6 per cent overall. These data are particularly relevant if considered as indicators of transport efficiency, since it is assumed that the higher the number of people who are accompanied on a private basis, the less effective is the transport network in responding to the needs of older people.

Satisfaction with the quality of public transport – frequency, comfort, hygiene, waiting and travelling times, costs and availability of information – is low among older people though it rises in older age groups. Among over 75 year olds, the rating of the number of bus stops, the availability and cleanliness of means of transport is very high, while widespread dissatisfaction lies with the high costs of public transport (SPI-CGIL/CER 1997: 135). It is evident that a policy aimed at improving older people's QoL in the transport sector should not only consider extending its network but also increasing its economic accessibility by offering cheaper fares to older people.

These data can be integrated with the results of a recent survey conducted in central Italy on a sample of 600 over 55 year olds, which confirmed the increased number of satisfied users among older age groups, but underlined the presence of several critical points (Marcellini *et al.* 1999: 88–103; ERC-ECMT 2000). One of these is the proportion of older people who are driven privately, which rises from 12 per cent of those between 65–74 to 27 per cent of the over eighties but, more importantly, the number of people who do not succeed in using the means of transport they need increases markedly in the older age groups, growing from almost nil in the 55–64 age group to 5 per cent among 75–79 year olds, to 17 per cent among people aged 80 and over. Among the possible reasons for this strong limitation of movement are the 'lack of comfort on buses' (complained about by 5 per cent of the people aged between 55–64, but by 66 per cent of those aged over 75), and the concurrence of several causes: 'too high bus steps' (54 per cent), 'low number of passengers who offer their seats to older people' (49 per cent), 'too few bus stops and shelters' (41 per cent), 'bus drivers' jerking when they start' (35 per cent) and 'low number of bus rides' (28 per cent).

New technologies

In Italy there is a widespread knowledge of the existence of new technologies but without corresponding use, and if this problem is not solved in today's informatics society, we run the risk of seeing a 'digital divide' (OECD 2001b), that is the rise of new forms of isolation and marginalization and consequently a deterioration of QoL among the less educated and poor especially older people (Palomba *et al.* 2001).

Television is without doubt the technology most widely used by older Italians (followed by the video recorder) (Palomba *et al.* 2001).[2] Among communication technologies the mobile phone is the most widely used. Italy is one of the European countries with the widest use of mobile phones (ESIS-ISPO 2000) and 25 per cent of older people own a mobile phone, with higher concentrations among men (33 per cent) and especially among those with monthly incomes higher than 2300 euros (65 per cent) (Palomba *et al.* 2001). Since mobile phones are often used by the whole family the rate of real users rises further, reaching almost 40 per cent of all families with at least one older person in it (Delai 1999: 50).

Answering machines are by comparison less common than mobile phones, since only 20 per cent of the people over 65 owns one while, among traditional household appliances, a dishwasher is present in 31 per cent of the households of the over 65s and the microwave oven, a late comer to Italy, only in 18 per cent of them (Palomba *et al.* 2001). One of the explanations for the low spread of the more complex household appliances is their high level of difficulty to use, due to the fact that instructions are often printed in a foreign language, the print is very small and difficult to read, or the language is often confusing (Delai 2000: 52).

Recent national surveys confirm that 20 per cent of the over 65s use an ATM card and about 6 per cent use credit cards, but these percentages drop to less than half among those over 75 and among women compared to men (Banca d'Italia 2000; ISTAT 2000a). The relatively scarce use of these technological instruments of payment among older Italians seems to depend on the fact that, although 53 per cent of them realize and acknowledge their usefulness, about 13 per cent consider them too complicated. In contrast automatic payment of bills through the bank is relatively more popular (32 per cent) (Palomba *et al.* 2001).

As for informatics and the use of PCs and the Internet, Italy lags behind other European countries (Kubitschke *et al.* 2002). Only 15 per cent of older Italians own a PC (20 per cent of men and 11 per cent of women), while a further 11 per cent would like to learn how to use one; 5 per cent have a subscription to the Internet, with a peak of 9 per cent in the age group between 60 and 64, which drops to 3 per cent in the 70–4 age group (Palomba *et al.* 2001). A survey carried out on the use of Italian Web sites devoted to the third age and on their use by older people has shown also that there is a difference in the approach to the computer society on the part of older Italians when compared with those in other countries (Luciani 1999, 2000). The Italian Web sites tend to be more static in the way they communicate or exchange news and focus on studies concerning old age; therefore, they do not succeed in creating a virtual community of people who can find a new social dimension on the Internet, as happens in other countries, particularly in North America. This situation is reflected by the small usage among the over 65s – who represent about 11 per cent of Internet users (CENSIS 2001) – and by the fact that the Web sites devoted to old age, despite their increasing number, only rarely represent the straightforward expression of an active involvement of the older population in the Internet (Luciani 1999). This is the case with the Web sites created by older people's associations (31 per cent) and by the Universities of the Third Age (16 per cent) to advertise their organizations, but the majority of the Web sites actually address older people as prospective users of the services they offer, most of which consist of telematics projects (10 per cent), travel and holidays (8 per cent), older people's homes (6 per cent) and various other fields of activity (30 per cent).

Despite this less than dynamic profile a recent national survey foresees that it will be older people who, in the future, will mostly increase the 'Web community' (Grillo 2001). This is due to the fact that many older people who are isolated or have mobility problems, could take advantage of the use of the Web to get information about a wide range of services. The attainment of this target would also overcome the risk of a digital divide, but requires the teaching of the basics necessary to use computers and the elimination of some obstacles, such as the relatively high costs of Web connection and of the necessary hardware and software, as well as training for their appropriate use.

Although the euro is not a new technology this change in the currency involves many basic aspects of daily life, and it is therefore important to observe how older people are facing this transformation. In 1998 the European Community Household Panel survey inserted some questions about the introduction of the euro (ISTAT 1999b).[3] At that time, the over 65s were less informed (77 per cent) than the younger age groups (95 per cent), their information being mainly drawn from the TV and the radio (97 per cent), and less often derived from either members of the family (40 per cent) or from friends and acquaintances (33 per cent). Housewives and retired people were those who expressed the highest degree of dissatisfaction with the quality of information received from the radio and the TV, which was considered poor or inadequate in almost one-third of the cases. Some older Italians, especially in the rural areas of the South still refer to their family network, where they exist, to use the new currency. This is in line with what a recent Eurobarometer survey has confirmed in terms of lower attachment and support of the older generations towards the new European currency (Eurobarometer 2003: B.61–64), although Italians in general are among the countries with the highest proportion of population with positive feelings towards it.

Physical and mental health functioning

In the country with the world's highest ratio between the number of medical doctors and the population (OECD 2000), the large number of studies that base their approach to QoL in old age mainly on health is no surprise. Though health represents one of the central aspects in the last phase of an individual's life (EURISPES 1993; SPI-CGIL 1997; CNEL 2000), the importance given to this dimension in Italy often tends to confine to the background the role played by other dimensions of life, which should all be integrated in a comprehensive approach. This is why this section of the chapter will focus mainly on the distinction between 'objective' and 'individually perceived' health status. By 'objective' health status we generally mean the results of clinical diagnoses derived from medical check ups carried out with a view to analysing the incidence of chronic degenerative pathologies and disabilities. By 'individually perceived' health status we mean the subjective evaluation of one's own health conditions, as they are experienced by the individual. The latter is considered to be an important variable to determine the level of a person's QoL, and at the same time one of the main indicators of the demand for health and social care (Presidenza del Consiglio dei Ministri 2000: 82). This is particularly true for older people, among whom a negative perception of health conditions has proved to be a highly reliable indicator of a frequent use of health services (Zuliani 2000: 4).

The two most important studies carried out in Italy on older people's health (Presidenza del Consiglio dei Ministri 2000) are the Italian Longitudinal Study on Ageing (ILSA), the first of its kind in the country, which uses medical diagnoses to assess objectively the incidence of chronic degenerative pathologies and disabilities among older people (IRP-CNR 1997); and a survey periodically carried out by ISTAT, which uses subjective health evaluations made by the older people interviewed, and their knowledge of the presence/absence of chronic diseases or disabilities (ISTAT 2001b).[4]

The results of these two surveys have not always been consistent, which demonstrates the gap between 'objective' and subjective assessments of health conditions. In particular, the ILSA study shows a greater spread of multiple pathologies at all ages, compared to the ISTAT survey (Presidenza del Consiglio dei Ministri 2000). This divergence between the high presence of pathologies and the individual's subjective health can be explained by the fact that pathologies characterized by no symptoms (such as hypertension) are often neither perceived nor diagnosed, and do not necessarily imply a worsening in the individual's subjective health.

The 'subjective health self-perception' analysed by the ISTAT survey allows us to obtain an overall evaluation of people's health, in order to determine the prevalence of poor health (of people who declare they are ill), of chronic patients (people who declare they suffer from at least one chronic disease) and of disabled people (those who experience serious difficulty in at least one of the activities of daily living (ADL)). The percentage of people who feel in good health steadily decreases with age, especially among the over 75s (Table 3.4, col. 1). Within this general trend, common to both sexes, women in all age groups say they feel in good health less frequently than men.

The number of people who suffer from chronic diseases appears to follow the opposite trend, increasing with age, and this also affects women particularly (col. 2–3). Moreover, because of the absence of diagnosis for many conditions, these data are underestimated. Many people declare themselves to be in good

Table 3.4 Self-perceived health conditions and chronic diseases among over 55 year olds, 2000 (per 100 persons of same age and sex)

Age group	1 In good health (a).		2 With at least one chronic disease (b).		3 With at least two chronic diseases (b).		4 Chronic patients in good health (c).	
	M	F	M	F	M	F	M	F
55–59	66.3	59.9	53.1	57.9	23.1	34.6	52.7	47.6
60–64	59.4	47.3	62.3	66.9	31.0	46.1	47.8	37.2
65–74	43.4	37.2	74.5	77.9	46.5	58.7	32.3	29.9
75 and over	28.2	23.6	82.7	85.0	60.6	69.3	21.9	19.1

Notes:
(a): per cent of persons who answered 'well' or 'very well' to the question 'how is your health?'
(b): per 100 persons
(c): per 100 persons suffering from at least one chronic disease
Source: ISTAT (2001b).

health even when affected by one or more chronic diseases (col. 4). This suggests that 'feeling well' for older people does not necessarily imply the absence of chronic conditions. Thus, beyond a certain age, people tend to consider 'normal' the presence of certain pathologies, of course provided these do not interfere too much with their normal daily activities.

This suggests that in order to connect adequately QoL and health conditions it is necessary to evaluate the impact that a deterioration of the latter exerts on the daily life of older people, keeping in mind that the presence of disabilities (as measured by ADLs) is much less widespread than chronic diseases in all age groups (Presidenza del Consiglio dei Ministri 2000). A more systematic use of this approach, which is more practical and more directly linked to several aspects of QoL, would lead to a better understanding of what seems to be one of the major concerns of older people, that is not so much the fear of 'diseases', but rather the fear of 'being forced to give up autonomy' (SPI-CGIL 1997).

The data provided by the ESAW project reveal that older Italians report on average a higher number of chronic conditions, use of medications and a worse quality of vision and hearing, but also less risky behaviour in terms of alcohol and tobacco consumption, than people of the same age living in Northern European countries (Ferring *et al.* 2003b: 19–40). This study confirms the existence of a similar, strong cross-national association between income and health status: older people with low income being over-represented in the cluster of persons in bad health (and vice versa). Older Italians seem to report much more frequently than other Europeans that they 'feel subjectively bad' when their objective status (in terms of number of disabling conditions, medications/prosthetics used and ADL-IADL status) is relatively good, and vice versa (Ferring *et al.* 2003b: 48–51). This is particularly relevant in the light of the other main result emerging from the ESAW study, showing that health status, together with material security, represents one of the two dimensions that mostly affect wellbeing in older Europeans, although in the Italian ESAW sample social support resources have an even stronger impact on life satisfaction (Chapter 8) (Ferring *et al.* 2003a: 25).

The ESAW survey produced interesting findings concerning mental health (Weber *et al.* 2003: 29–31). Based on the Mental Health Scale used by Fillenbaum and colleagues for the OARS (Older Americans' Resources and Services) study, which is made of 10 dichotomous items on symptoms like restlessness, worrying, depressed mood and drive, energy, interests, sleep, paranoia and loneliness (Fillenbaum 1988), ESAW data show for older Italians the worst overall results, although not significantly dissimilar from those recorded for Sweden and Luxembourg (Weber *et al.* 2003: 29–31). A clear correlation has been found between mental health and *age*, with increasingly worse levels of mental health in older cohorts (but not in all ESAW countries); *gender*, older women showing worse levels than men (in a more pronounced way than in other countries); *living arrangements*, older people living alone recording worse scores; as well as *working conditions*, the employed reporting higher levels of mental health (although not so pronounced as in other countries).

Employment, early retirement and material security

Employment plays a major role, although not comparable to the influence of health, in determining the QoL of older people: it determines the amount of the pension that will be received after retirement and it influences the general economic conditions and lifestyle developed throughout the life course.

Work is currently one of the main worries of Italians over the age of 50 (CNEL 2000: 4). This reflects the steep decline of employment among older workers, especially among men (Cataldi and Ricci 2000), over the last few decades and this can also be observed in the great majority of European countries (Walker 1997: 17–19).

Given this situation it is necessary to consider some aspects that characterize Italy when compared to other countries:

- pre-retirement, although officially abandoned at the moment, has been frequent until recently (Tronti 1998), owing to a government policy that allowed
the early retirement of civil workers and used pre-retirement as a social 'shock
absorber' in order to soften the impact of the economic crisis in the private
sector, with the effect of producing a large number of relatively young retirees;

- due to the young age of many retired persons, the phenomenon of working
after retirement is quite widespread (Geroldi 2000), and this has been
further encouraged by the recent abolition under the Financial Law (2002)
of the ban on combining a pension and earnings (Law no. 448/2001);

- older people in Italy, although remaining one of the groups most exposed
to the risk of poverty, appear to be relatively privileged, compared to their
European counterparts, due to family solidarity and resource redistribution
within the family network, and also in comparison to the high unemployment
rates among young people (Frey 1999; Frey and Livraghi 1999; De Vincenti
2000; Frey 2000a; De Vincenti and Rodano 2001).

Economic circumstances

As a consequence of the income drop due to retirement, older people generally
represent one of the groups most frequently at risk of poverty, which in
turn represents one of the major threats to QoL in old age. Cross-national
studies, however, show that this risk might be less prominent in Italy than in
other European countries, due to a more age-balanced income distribution
(De Vincenti 2000: 82–112). In Italy the percentage of older people who have
an income under the poverty threshold (below 50 per cent of the average per
capita income) is much lower than in Germany or in the UK (Table 3.5).

The fact that the equation 'old person = low income' is less applicable in Italy
than in other countries can be explained by several factors, among which three
play a major role. First of all, the trend to start a new career after retirement
represents a positive factor because many 'young' retired people can now add
the income of new employment to their pension. Secondly, there is an 'income
re-distributive mediation role' played by the family that is much more evident
than in Northern European countries and means older people receive intergenerational income flows from other members of the (extended) family (OECD
2001a: 16). At the same time, older people often help other members of their
families financially, particularly in southern Italy (SPI-CGIL 1997). Thirdly,
older people have a relatively strong inclination to save (Frey 2001b: 5). This is
mirrored by particularly careful behaviour in terms both of expenditure and of

Table 3.5 Percentage of over 65 year old population and of retired persons in condition of poverty in Italy, UK and Germany (1990–1993, percentage values on total numbers of families)

	Italy	United Kingdom	Germany
Total population	23.6	26.9	21.3
by age group:			
– population aged 66–75	22.1	40.5	32.1
– over 75 year old population	30.0	56.2	45.8
by prevalent source of income:			
– pension	16.4	40.3	29.9
– subordinate work	11.3	5.1	5.9
– self-employed work	18.0	8.0	4.7

Source: De Vincenti (2000).

types of goods purchased in that older people have a lower propensity to purchase non-essential goods and a higher propensity to purchase primary goods and services (ISTAT 1997: 59–60), such as rent, fuel, electric power and health expenses (Presidenza del Consiglio dei Ministri 2000: 62).

Furthermore, there is house ownership. In Italy 80 per cent of men over 75 and 73 per cent of women over 75 live in owner-occupied houses, compared with 71 per cent and 61 per cent respectively of people under 59 years of age (ISTAT 1997: 64–5). The ESAW research study shows that only 7 per cent of older Italians are still repaying a mortgage on their home, in contrast to other Europeans for whom the proportion is over 20 per cent (Lamura *et al.* 2003: 27).

The present situation is the result of a substantial improvement of the living standards of older people which has characterized the last few years, at least until the introduction of the euro. Between 1989 and 1998 the individual income of people over 65 increased by 74 per cent, in comparison with an increase of just 14 per cent among those under 30 years old, who are the group with the lowest individual income (Banca d'Italia 2000). A direct consequence of this improvement is that, over the same period of time, the number of families with an older person whose income is lower than 10,000 euros has fallen from 56.7 per cent to 29.8 per cent, while the number of those whose income is between 10,000 and 20,000 euros has increased from 30.1 per cent to 42.6 per cent (Presidenza del Consiglio dei Ministri 2000: 65–7).

However, the risk of poverty is not equally distributed among older people and there are some categories whose incomes are lower than those in other countries (Frey 2002: 5). Older people who live alone, for instance, are much more at risk in Italy than in other countries, and families whose 'family head' is an older woman are poorer, since women generally receive lower pensions than men, either because they usually retire earlier than men or because they live on survivorship annuities. Furthermore, the proportion of income derived from work tends to be much lower for women than for men over 60 (2.4 per cent compared with 12.6 per cent) (ISTAT 1997: 58–9), whereas the risk of poverty is small among families where the 'family head' is a retired man.

Hard data such as income level, house ownership and other similar indicators are not sufficient to explain the possible impact exerted by material security on subjective life satisfaction, and this is probably even more so in the case of older people. The ESAW study has pointed out that a more comprehensive indicator could possibly be provided by the perceived adequacy of available material resources to one's needs, an item (called material or economic adequacy) that directly reflects the ability of one's resources to meet one's specific needs, thus relating material security strongly with wellbeing (Lamura *et al.* 2003: 40–5). According to these findings, older Italians report the lowest levels of material adequacy in Europe, particularly among women, older age groups and less educated groups in rural areas.

Employment

Compared to the European average, the activity rate of the older Italian population is quite low, for men especially in the 50–9 age group, while among women this happens for virtually all age groups. The only exception to this general tendency is represented by the activity rate of men over 65, which is slightly higher than the European average, due to the presence of a relatively high number of self-employed workers in the service sector.

The low male activity rate in the 50–9 age group depends on the presence of early retired people, which is strongly linked to the early retirement policy adopted until recently in some sectors of private industry hit by the economic crisis, as well as to the regular retirement of a substantial number of workers who had started work at a relatively young age (between 15 and 20 years). The relatively high activity rate of men over 65 represents the consequence of the important role played by the services sector in Italy through a widespread network of small retail shops, in many cases run on a family basis, which, due to the flexible organization of working times, are suited to older people (Romano and Sgritta 2000). Partly, however, work in old age can also be explained by the need to earn more (because of low retirement pensions), especially among some categories of self-employed people (for example craftsmen). As for the low rates of women's participation in the labour market, this is mainly due to the higher number of housewives than in other European countries, and only marginally to the presence of young retired female workers who, in the public sector until recently, could retire after just 14 years and six months if they were working mothers (Miniati 2000).

In Italy improving QoL for older workers means intervening in two main fields: on the one hand, improving the requalification and professional training of workers over 50, in order to avoid their early retirement or dismissal from the labour force (Eurolink Age 2000); on the other hand, given the presence of a high number of young retired workers, preventing 'ageist' attitudes towards those who wish to continue working after retirement (Miniati 2000). In fact the oldest age groups are more favourable to a policy of labour market liberalization in terms of recruitment and dismissals, and advocate measures to raise retirement age (CNEL 2000; Delai 2001).

Early retirement

In order to understand the Italian case concerning early retirement and its consequences in terms of QoL in old age, reference is necessary to two peculiar aspects of the labour market and the pension system. First of all, in Italy the term 'unemployment' is associated mainly with younger people (who experience much higher rates than any other European country, reaching 30 per cent for young men under 25 and 40 per cent for women under 25, with peaks up to 50 per cent in the south of the country), while unemployment rates for people between 50 and 64 years old are quite low for both sexes, and definitely lower than the European average (Cataldi and Ricci 2000: 71). Secondly, Italy is the European country with the lowest retirement age, varying normally between 57 and 65 (compared with a 60–7 range in the other European countries), but even lower in case of a contribution period of at least 40 years (De Vincenti 2000). This last aspect, together with the frequent resort to early retirement until just a few years ago, explains why Italy spends a much higher percentage of its GDP on retirement pensions than the other OECD countries (Carbonin 1997: 91; OECD 2001a: 82–4),[5] which some proposals currently under discussion in the Italian Parliament aim to reduce through an increase in the retirement age up to 68 years and/or the introduction of incentives in favour of workers who decide not to retire and to work longer (Law no. 448/2001).

The average retirement age is 59.6 for men and 55.9 for women (Palomba *et al.* 2001), while the number of people who retire under 50 is quite substantial (Sgritta and Saporiti 1997). This means that Italian workers retire on average three or four years before those in other OECD countries and that, given the current life expectancy, they will receive pensions for about 21 years (compared with 17.8 in other OECD countries) and for more than 26 years in the case of women (compared with 23 years of the other OECD countries) (OECD 2001a).

Given the peculiarity of this situation it is very surprising that this topic is considerably under-researched in terms of the consequences of early retirement on the QoL of older people. One exception is represented by the studies carried out by Mirabile and colleagues (1998) who, having reviewed the Italian literature, point out that there exists among workers, especially at the lower occupational levels, a sort of defensive attitude, which shows that early retirement is experienced as an opportunity for a new career only by a small proportion of workers, while its negative connotation of dismissal from work prevails among the majority.

Work after retirement

A phenomenon that has been studied systematically only in recent years is the so-called second career, where people after retirement take up a new job or become *de facto* self-employed. For several years, the number of retired people who continue working after retirement has been increasing, often as consultants for their previous employers, thus in a role that is different from that typical of an employee or of a self-employed person (Mirabile and Carrera 1999). According to the latest available data, at the beginning of 1998 the number of retired people who had started a new career, mainly men (69 per cent) and concentrated in northern Italy (60 per cent), amounted to almost 900,000 people, that is about 7–8 per cent of the total retired population, with a peak of 17 per cent in the age group between 50 and 54 (Geroldi 2000). Thus a large number of workers, with the complicity of the peculiar Italian pension system, adopt an explicit income strategy aimed at early retirement followed by new employment on a more independent and flexible basis.

Very few studies have examined the motivations behind this trend, but it has been observed that the average pension of those who start a new career is slightly higher than average and this trend is more common in northern Italy (Geroldi 2000: 88). It can be inferred, therefore, that the main motivation for this behaviour might not be the low amount of the retirement pension but rather the opportunity to combine it with a work activity that is more conducive to a new phase of life, and at the same time more appreciated by many employers.

The ESAW study confirms the significance of the working retirees in the Italian labour market, where they comprise almost one-third of the active population in the age group 60–9 (Lamura *et al.* 2003: 22), a level that is much higher than that in other European countries. Furthermore, working retirees have on average a higher life satisfaction than other retirees of the same age, suggesting that this active approach to the retirement life phase can positively affect one's wellbeing, unless this work is not a freely chosen option but is dictated by economic constraints.

The perception of retirement

People who are still employed identify the most important changes when retirement comes as the opportunity to live with 'less stress' (28 per cent), but also the fear of marginality and passivity characterized by feelings of 'boredom, loneliness and uselessness' (25 per cent). A similar percentage of workers (24 per cent) think that retirement will be an opportunity to 'enjoy life and have fun' or to devote more time to the 'home and to family and social relations' (23 per cent). The answers are not significantly gender specific but reflect the education, professional status and residential area of the respondents (Palomba *et al.* 2001).

Among those who have already retired two main aspects can be distinguished: the most important changes that occurred in the retired person's life after retirement and the presence of possible regrets due to the fact that retired people miss their jobs. On the first point, the number of retirees saying that the most important change after retirement is 'more time for the care of the home and for social and family relations' is almost double that of the working population (44 per cent versus 23 per cent). Fewer than expected (22 per cent versus 25 per cent) are retirees who experience negative aspects such as a feeling of 'more loneliness and boredom' or 'of being old and useless', whereas a wider gap resulted between those who state they feel 'less stressed' (18 per cent versus 28 per cent) or have 'more time to enjoy themselves' (15 per cent versus 24 per cent). Overall, therefore, retirement is associated with a greater engagement with families and social relations than was supposed before entering it, with fewer opportunities for rest and enjoyment than they expected and a negative experience of loneliness, boredom or futility that affects more than one retiree out of five.[6]

Some important differences emerge owing to different models of participation in the labour market on the part of men and women belonging to the cohort born in the 1930s, as well as to territorial variations, in terms of different work typologies, career opportunities and the value attributed to work itself. In particular, retired men more often feel 'less stress' and have 'more time to enjoy themselves', especially if they are educated (at a degree or diploma level), if they live in the central or northern regions of Italy (probably because of a more stressful work rhythm of the big- and medium-sized industries of these regions) and if they have not been retired long. Retired women, on the contrary, signal as by far the most important change in their life habits having 'more time for the home and for social relations' but also the feeling of 'deep loneliness and boredom' that makes them feel 'old and purposeless'. These latter answers are more typical also among people with a low education level (elementary school), people living in central-southern Italy and those who have been retired for a long period. Furthermore, with advancing age, there is an increase in the percentage of men and women describing retirement as 'passivity and marginality', which probably reflects age and the type of socialization of the respondents.

As for the presence of possible 'regrets in terms of missing one's previous job', 58 per cent of the retirees declare they do not miss it at all, and an even higher percentage (76 per cent) state that, had they been given the opportunity, they would have preferred not to work at all. There is a remarkable divide between reality and expectations here, because the proportion of working people who believe they will not miss their work once they are retired is only 31 per cent, thus showing a concern among workers about their life after retirement.

Gender is important in the approach to retirement. Focusing only on employed persons, 37 per cent of working women think they will miss the relational and social aspects of their job, such as the 'relationship with their colleagues and contact with people', whereas 23 per cent declare they will miss the routine, such as 'leaving home in the morning' and 'their job daily commitments'. The concern about these apparently marginal and routine aspects of work might be explained by the fact that work has represented, for many women of this generation, an achievement and a way to escape from the limitations of domestic life. As for men, the prevailing attitude is that they will miss 'nothing' (33 per cent), or that they will miss the 'expressive' aspects of work, such as 'learning new things', 'feeling useful', or, in the case of 15 per cent (as opposed to 8 per cent of women), they will resent losing the economic aspect of work, which is 'higher income'. Finally, the difference between the percentage of men (21 per cent) and women (5 per cent) who regret losing the feeling of being useful is likely to depend on the fact that women of the older generations are traditionally and culturally more ready than men to be useful within the family.

Conclusion

The information reported in this chapter shows that housing plays a major role for the QoL of older Italians – also in association with the relatively low rate of institutionalization – but this mainly concerns the private sphere. Public policy on housing is marginal in Italy, with negative consequences for the safety level of many dwellings. While the use of transportation and new technologies in older age seem to represent less important issues in the public debate, health-related topics are central, to the point that one might speak of the 'medicalization' of old age in Italy. Finally, from an economic point of view, a further peculiarity of Italy is the presence of a relatively large number of retired people, due to the past generosity of the early retirement system, which allows many Italian retirees to keep on working in a 'second career', thus contributing to a reduced risk of poverty among older Italians compared with other Europeans, which also stems from the redistribution effect of the family networks, which are analysed in Chapter 8.

Notes

1. Franci's work has shown that the pleasantness of the rooms, the quality of food and the high professional competence of the staff can significantly influence the level of satisfaction of older people living in institutions.

2. This survey – to which most data reported in this paragraph refer – was carried out in 1999 on a sample of over 4300 persons between 60 and 74 years of age, stratified by sex, age and region of residence.

3. The ECHP is an annual survey begun in 1994, starting from a sample in 12 EU countries made up from 61,106 families and 127,000 individuals, of which 7989 families and 24,063 individuals resided in Italy.

4. The difference between the two studies is also a quantitative one because the ISTAT 'multipurpose surveys' reach a sample of about 60,000, which is representative of the whole Italian population, while the ILSA study is based on a non-random sample of about 6000 non-institutionalized elderly between 65 and 74 years of age, recruited through 213 clinical centres distributed throughout Italy.

5. Higher pension spending in Italy is partly explained by the fact that the total amount of public expenditure on social welfare is below the European average, and that the expenditure on pensions includes expenses that do not pertain to social security (Geroldi 2000: 179).

6. This study was not longitudinal and, therefore, it cannot state how much of these differences depend on a cohort effect (connected to a change in values between the various generations of retired people), how much is due to a more general transformation of the general historical and social milieu, and how much depends on the role change of the individual (from a working to a retired person).

4

The Netherlands: quality of life in old age I

Annemarie Peeters, Beitske Bouwman and
Kees Knipscheer

Introduction

On 1 January 2000 there were 3.7 million people aged 55 and over in the Netherlands, around 23 per cent of the total population. By comparison, in 1970 there were 2.5 million in this group and projections suggest that the figure will rise to around six million in 2030, a 63 per cent increase (SCP 2001).

Slightly more than half of the over-55s are women and roughly 30 per cent live alone (Table 4.1). The oldest age groups consist mainly of women, who account for 63 per cent of 75 to 84 year olds and 74 per cent of those aged over 85. The proportion of women in the higher age groups is expected to fall in the years ahead, owing to a reduction in the difference in life expectancy between men and women (Maas *et al.* 1997: 47). This decline may be attributed to the declining differences in smoking behaviour and working conditions (SER 1999).

The fact that the difference in average life expectancy between men and women is steadily shrinking does not necessarily mean that the proportion of single older people will also fall. According to forecasts by Statistics Netherlands (CBS), the percentage of older people living in a one-person household will remain roughly the same in the years ahead (De Beer, De Jong and Visser 1993; Knipscheer *et al.* 1995), at slightly under 30 per cent. Obviously, widowhood is not the only significant factor in this household form: people may be in a one-person household because of divorce, or may never have cohabited (SCP 2001).

A particularly large increase can be expected in the number of 55 to 64 year olds between 2005 and 2015, as a result of the 'baby boom' after the Second

Table 4.1 Some demographic characteristics of older people, 1 January 2000 (in absolute numbers × 1000 and percentages)

	55–64 years	65–74 years	75–84 years	> 85 years	Total
Older people (× 1000)	1582.9	1194.9	731.9	225.7	3735.3
Women (%)	50	54	63	74	55
One-person households (%)	16	28	51	72	29
Turkish, Moroccan, Surinamese and Antillean elderly (× 1000)	52.5	16.5	5.1a	a	74.2

Owing to the small numbers, the 75–84 year olds and over 85s have been combined
Source: SCP (2001).

World War. Not only will the number of older people increase, but future cohorts will also differ on a wide range of aspects from the present generation of older people. It is to be expected that, because of the increase in education level in connection with a relatively better financial position and health, in future older people will stay active longer and will place high demands on their life circumstances and QoL. Most of the data examined in this chapter were drawn from the SCP report on older people (2001) and from CBS data.

Definition and measurement of quality of life

The many attempts to clarify what QoL is about can be divided into three approaches (Maes and Petry 2000). Firstly, the 'objective approach' in which the sum of a series of objective measurable good life circumstances is at the centre. This approach looks at, for example, the labour market position and financial status, health, leisure activities, size and structure of the social network, opportunities and so on. Secondly, the 'subjective approach' assumes that one's QoL should be understood in terms of subjective feelings and experienced wellbeing and satisfaction with one's living situation. Thirdly, the 'interactive approach' adds another element, namely the degree of 'goodness-of-fit' between the person and his or her environment. Quality of life is considered optimal when someone has the opportunities to aim for and realize personal goals and when he or she has the capacity and support resources to meet the demands and expectations of the environment.

According to Tesch-Romer *et al.* (2001) QoL is a multidimensional concept and includes material and non-material, objective and subjective, and individual and collective aspects of wellbeing and welfare. Objective living conditions influence the agency of individuals and their ability to control their own environments. The subjective living experience, on the other hand, refers to the self-evaluations and feelings of the individuals. Within the domain of subjective wellbeing, several distinctions should be made. Not only general indicators (life satisfaction, happiness) but also domain-specific indicators should be considered. Cognitive judgements and emotional experiences can be distinguished within subjective wellbeing. Subjective wellbeing is not a single, bipolar dimension, but rather two independent dimensions of positive and negative affect that have to be considered separately. Finally, QoL should not only be considered by taking into account the perspective of the individual, but also the societal perspective: it is important to know what opportunities societies create for their members.

The CBS has made an inventory of key indicators of QoL in the Netherlands. It has compiled a large collection of key figures of the life situation of the population (and of specific groups within the population). It approaches the concept of QoL via indicators including demographic data, housing, environment, criminality and labour market position (CBS 2000). The SCP approaches the life situation of individuals – quality of existence – via the design of a life situation index (Figure 4.1). The focus is on items like health, mobility, housing situation, social participation, leisure activities, participation in sports, consumer durables and holidays. The index provides a way of organizing the many possible topics that are related to the concept of QoL (SCP 2001).

In this scheme a cause-effect relationship is assumed between resources and life situation: the more resources one has, the greater the chance of a good life situation. The actual situation someone is in is important but so are the values people give for (parts of) their life situation, and the extent of their happiness (SCP/SSN 2001).

Measurements

Dutch measurements of QoL among older people are scarce. The most commonly used are originally from other countries, such as the US and the UK, translated into Dutch and made suitable for use in the Netherlands. The most commonly used types of measure are those related to health and QoL from the medical sciences (Bogaerts, in press).

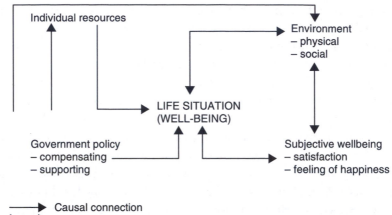

Individual resources
Education, work and income, self-support, age, household composition, ethnic-cultural origin and so on.

Environment
Correlation between physical quality and social characteristics such as: satisfaction of residents, criminality, composition of population.

Figure 4.1 Life situation index
Source: SCP (2001).

Quality of life of nursing home residents

This measurement defines QoL as: 'the opinion of older clients of nursing homes of the quality of sensory, physical, mental and social functioning and the experienced safety and autonomy'. Important factors are health status and the housing and care provided in a nursing home.

Rand-36

This measurement defines QoL as 'the perception of the physical, mental and social consequences of unhealthiness in daily life of individuals, is the basic assumption of the concept QoL'. This instrument measures general health status. Physical dimensions are physical functioning, role limitations, pain, and subjective evaluation of health. Psychosocial dimensions are vitality, social functioning and mental health.

GLAS (Groningen Longitudinal Ageing Study)

This study focuses on daily living, wellbeing and the need for care of older people rather than QoL as such. This is because of doubts about the measurement of the unclear and subjective concept of QoL and, specifically, which dimensions and domains are a part of it. The study uses different kinds of scales to measure physical wellbeing; social wellbeing; stimulation and comfort; status and affection; activities; endowments and resources.

SEIQoL (Schedule for the Evaluation of Individual Quality of Life)

The SeiQoL measures individual QoL. It originated in the UK and has been adapted for the Netherlands. Here QoL is measured from the perspective of older people. The individual nominates five determinants that are important to his or her QoL. Indicators are: family; hobby; health; social contacts; religion; environment; marriage; mobility; independence; and financial status.

All instruments mentioned above use scales and questionnaires with various dimensions and domains, except the SEIQoL, which takes the perception of the individual as the point of departure (Schölzel-Dorenbos 2000).

Environments of ageing

Housing

Despite the fact that government policy in the Netherlands has for some time focused on encouraging independent living and changing from institutionalized to semi-institutionalized and community-based provision, a relatively high proportion of older people still live in institutions. The central objective of the policy on housing and care is to offer optimal choices for people with a degree of care (for example for older people) and increase the quality of care and housing. The aim is to increase independence and self-reliance of people in all age brackets for as long as possible (Zorgnota 2002: 80).

Until recently older people with an increasing need for care were forced to move. Now it is increasingly assumed that even when the level of frailty increases people can still stay in their own home (Mulder 2001). Since 1 April 1994 home adaptations have been partly funded by the Services for the Disabled Act (WVG).

Older people living independently

Currently roughly 92 per cent of the over-65s live independently (Ministerie van VROM 2000; Mulder 2001; SCP 2001). Two-thirds of the over-55s live in a single family dwelling; the rest occupy flats. If the total older population is subdivided by age and household composition, it becomes apparent that single people more often live in flats than multi-person households, although the proportion of the latter category living in a flat increases with age. People aged over 75, by contrast, are less likely to live in a single-family dwelling; this group often live in a flat with a lift.

The quality of housing for older people has improved slightly for several reasons. In the first place, the proportion of older people in recently built accommodation has increased, particularly among the over-75s. This is because of the construction of dwellings specifically aimed at older people. Second, the amount of space in the homes of older people has increased. The proportion of older people living in one and two rooms has fallen in recent years while the proportion living in large dwellings with five or more rooms has increased. An increase in the surface area of the accommodation also appears to have contributed to the improvement in the quality of older people's housing. The percentage with a relatively small living room fell markedly, while the percentage with a larger living room increased sharply over the same period.

The Dutch welfare society is not static. Older people opt increasingly for independent living with customized care in their own home or in housing care complexes (providing a combination of housing and care) (Teng 2001). Where home adaptation is not possible or where help is needed close at hand, older people often decide to move into a more sheltered form of housing offering a combination of housing and care. The housing care complex (*wozoco*), combining housing and care services, is a phenomenon firmly rooted in the 1990s. (The care centre and sheltered housing schemes date from previous decades.) The average number of homes per complex was considerably lower in the 1990s than the preceding period, indicating a reduction in the construction of new sheltered housing complexes. The majority of dwellings, 69 per cent, are close to a residential care home; 9 per cent are situated near a service centre and 10 per cent close to some other form of service provision facility; but 12 per cent of the homes are not close to any other provision (SCP 2001).

Physical and social aspects of the neighbourhood

The neighbourhood can be considered in terms of its physical aspects (residential setting, parking spaces, public transport and so on) and social aspects (individuals' subjective perceptions of the neighbourhood, including the residents, nuisance and safety). In general older people are considerably more satisfied with the physical aspects of their residential setting than younger people. Older people are also more content with their residential setting in general and experience less nuisance from odour, dust, noise or traffic than the younger age group. This pattern of a satisfaction level that increases with age also occurs within the older population: the over-75s have fewer problems with their residential setting than the 'younger old'. These differences between the age groups are less clear cut when it comes to the level of amenities in the neighbourhood. In fact, older people feel more often than younger people that there are too few shops in the neighbourhood and insufficient public transport. Older people also complain more than younger people about the lack of parking spaces and the absence of green spaces. The differences within the older population are low.

Older people are generally satisfied with their homes and residential setting, although they do relatively frequently feel unsafe: fears of being robbed or accosted are common, especially among older people living alone, many of whom are women. These feelings derive in part from the fact that a residential setting is unsafe or perceived to be unsafe. Simple measures can often resolve this situation, for example, talking to the other residents of a neighbourhood (possibly with the help of a neighbourhood survey) has been tried with success in many places. Although few older people dislike living in their neighbourhood, and few of them do not feel at home there, one in three say that they do not feel any particular ties to their own neighbourhood (SCP 2001: 294).

Residential and nursing homes

Roughly 5 per cent of the over-65s live in residential homes and approximately 2 per cent in nursing homes. In total, around 160,000 older people (aged over 65) live in such an institution. These are mainly the very elderly: more than 80,000 people living in a care or nursing home are aged 85 or over (Ministerie van VROM 2000; Mulder 2001; SCP 2001). There has been a marked reduction in scale in residential care homes in recent years, with the average number of beds/living units and residents being much smaller in recently built homes than in older facilities. Older people needing a degree of care (social and/or physical) live in residential care homes, while those with serious somatic and/or psychosomatic problems are housed in nursing homes (Table 4.2). The most important reason given for moving to a residential care home is the heavy burden of running the household. Another key factor affecting this decision is when home care services and/or family and friends are no longer able to meet the need for care. Furthermore, health fears play an important role for single people: they are afraid that something will go wrong when there is no one around. A decision to move to a nursing home is based to an even greater extent on the need for care; 70 per cent of nursing home residents state that home care services and friends and family were unable to offer sufficient care, prompting the move to a nursing home (Table 4.2).

Table 4.2 Housing characteristics of residents of residential care homes or nursing homes 2000 (%)

	Residential care homes				Nursing homes			
	65–74 yrs	75–84 yrs	> 85 yrs	Total	65–74 yrs	75–84 yrs	> 85 yrs	Total
Dissatisfied with number of rooms	29	28	29	28				
Dissatisfied with area of dwelling	32	22	25	24				
Living space								
One room alone					26	30	24	27
One room shared with another person					30	34	31	32
One room shared with 2–3 persons					26	19	17	20
One room shared with 4–5 persons					18	17	28	21
Opinion of own space (people who do not have their own room)								
Own space is sufficient					48	41	52	47
Would like to share with fewer people					19	10	20	15
Would like to have own room					34	49	28	38
Reasons for moving to home**								
Public home care services can't offer necessary care	42	39	35	37	65	74	72	71
Family etc. unable to offer necessary care	35	40	36	37	59	70	79	70

(Running) the household became too burdensome	60	58	57	57	70	64	62	65
Health fears if no-one is around	31	41	40	40	39	44	32	39
Alone in former home and wanted more contact	20	13	12	13	11	17	15	15
Former home unsuitable, impractical or too expensive	17	20	21	20	31	26	15	24
Former neighbourhood too unsafe	11	2	4	4	3	0	2	1
Pressure from others	34	41	42	41	37	38	44	40

** Question only put to those approached directly, mainly in somatic departments

Percentage indicating that a reason was a key factor in their decision to move

Source: SCP (2001); SCP (OII2000).

There has been a marked reduction in scale in residential care homes, but the amount of space per living unit has increased sharply in recent years. This trend appears to meet the residents' desire for more living space. A third of care home residents are dissatisfied with the number of rooms they have at their disposal, while between a quarter and a third feel their living unit is too small. The number of complaints about the size of units in which people live is considerably smaller in recently built homes than in older complexes. Even more than in the case of residential care homes, residents of nursing homes are clearly dissatisfied with their own living space. Fewer than half those residents who do not have their own room are satisfied on this point; almost 40 per cent of them would like their own room, while 15 per cent would like to share a room with fewer people. Thus not having one's own room in an institution is no longer acceptable today (SCP 2001).

Transport

Mobility is seen as a right in the Netherlands. It is a necessary condition to realize self-reliance and to participate in social activities. Slightly more than half of the over-65s households own a car and 15 per cent of the over-70s have a driving licence. The use of bus/tram or underground increases with age but is a relatively small user group (6 per cent of respondents) compared to the car (41 per cent) according to figures of the General Netherlands Federation of Older People (ANBO 2001). Limitations in walking are common in people aged over 65 and they comprise half of those who have problems with public transport.

Collective transport is provided for disabled older people and others who have difficulties using public transport. The Services for the Disabled Act (WVG) gave local authorities responsibility for the delivery of transport services and wheelchairs. Roughly two-thirds of the individual transport facilities and wheelchairs are being allocated to people aged over 65, who account for approximately 75 per cent of newly allocated entitlements to collective transport (SCP 2001; Ipso Facto and SGBO 2001). A survey by Ipso Facto of 319 collective transport clients shows that people are generally very satisfied with the WVG provisions. The greatest dissatisfactions concern not knowing how long a journey will last and having to wait. One of the problems with collective transport cited by users relates to long-distance transport. The government assumes that people, including those with functional impairments, will use public transport for this. However, because this service is insufficiently accessible a new travel service, Traxx, was introduced on 1 July 1999. This system makes use of the existing transport facilities, such as train and collective transport, combined with additional services, for example for transfers. Disabled people can travel via Traxx at the normal public transport fares.

Those taking advantage of WVG provisions were asked to what extent they themselves considered that the Act had an impact on their independence. They stated above all that these provisions enabled them to feel better in themselves and less dependent on others (approximately 80 per cent). The effect on their ability to continue living independently or to participate in community activities was slightly less pronounced, although two-thirds of users still believed that the Act helped them in this respect, too. Older people felt, to a slightly lesser extent than younger users, that the Act had an impact on the way in which they were able to perform their daily activities or to participate in the community. People in severe need of help took a slightly more positive view than others on a number of points concerning the effect of the Act; for example, thanks to the WVG they felt less dependent on others than people requiring little help. Roughly a third of users said they were completely independent of others thanks to their WVG provisions; these were people with transport provisions. Wheelchair users were also largely independent of others thanks to their WVG provision.

Use of technology

Older people are the most disadvantaged group in the information society. Almost half of them experience problems in using equipment or machines. Research by Freudenthal (1999) suggests that there are problems with equipment design, including legibility of screens and labels, use of a foreign language, programming and motor control during operation. Manuals frequently create problems: they are often too thick, or too thin, are unclear and poorly formulated, the font size is often too small or the foreign language inaccessible. Older people are one of the groups who are at a disadvantage as regards ownership and use of modern ICT products (Van Dijk *et al.* 2000). The over-65s, in particular, own considerably less ICT products than younger people, and ownership levels among the over-75s are even lower than among 65 to 74 year olds. PC ownership depends partly on income, education level, household composition and gender. These differences can also be observed within age categories; older people with a high income and high education level are more likely to have a PC than their less well off and less well educated peers. The differences between the sexes are relatively small.

However, the most important influence on the age differences in both ownership and usage has to do with whether or not people possess the necessary computer skills, which is much more important than education level, income or work experience. Older people require computer training above all in order to enable them to begin using computers. Today's young senior citizens much more often own and use a PC than the over-65s (Table 4.3). They also regularly come into contact with PCs at work and acquire computer skills.

There are currently many places where older people can follow courses, such as community centres, regional training centres or welfare centres for older people. People who do not have access to modern ICT resources at home need not be excluded from the information society; access can also be obtained at other locations, for example in libraries, Internet cafes, community centres. Many older people still harbour a disinterest in ICT and possibly also a fear of the computer, but it is to be expected that older people will increasingly find their way into the digital world in the future (SCP 2001).

Physical and mental health

Government policy documents on the future of healthcare in the Netherlands consistently talk about the burden that will be placed on the system owing to the increase in the number of older people. These statements are based on three observations. The first is that old age often brings with it infirmities, and that an increase in the number of older people will therefore automatically lead to an increase in the number of ill and vulnerable Dutch citizens. Secondly, the Dutch regard good health as a great asset and (older) Dutch citizens do not like ill health, and place high demands on the healthcare system. Thirdly, the Dutch constitution stipulates that caring for the health of the population is a task of the government; this means that the government has to a certain extent undertaken to meet the high standards set by the ageing population (SCP 2001). The trend in the health status of the Dutch population depends on many factors and personal characteristics. In addition to age these include socio-economic status, genetic factors, living situation and lifestyle characteristics, personality and external circumstances. According to the definition applied by the World Health Organization (WHO), health is regarded not only as absence of illness, but also a general feeling of wellbeing (SCP 2001).

Physical health

The life expectancy of men is 75 years, that of women almost 81 years (SCP 2001). According to the LASA study[1], most of these years of life will be spent in perceived good health. A characteristic of the health status of older people is

Table 4.3 Presence and use of a personal computer, laptop or notebook in households 1999 (%)

	Presence				Use			
	35–54 yrs	55–64 yrs	65–74 yrs	≥75 yrs	35–54 yrs	55–64 yrs	65–74 yrs	≥75 yrs
Men	78	54	29	11	63	41	18	8
Women	75	41	18	6	48	21	7	3
Primary/lower secondary education	67	37	17	5	43	20	8	3
Upper secondary education	83	60	35	8	63	43	19	6
Higher education	93	82	46	27	79	64	32	20
Low income	47	23	12	4	32	14	7	3
Middle income	74	46	22	11	53	31	11	7
High income	89	73	41	14	68	52	25	7
One-person household	49	29	10	4	58	32	14	6
Multi-person household	80	51	28	12	41	23	7	3

Source: SCP (2001).

that increasing age leads to a gradual increase in chronic health complaints, ultimately accompanied by long-term functional limitations and the decline, although not the disappearance, of acute health problems (Deeg *et al.* 2000; Verbrugge 1995). More than half the 'young old' (65 to 74 years) and almost two-thirds of the very elderly have one or more chronic disorders. Among the over-80s, however, 38 per cent report that they suffer from none of these ill-nesses. The most common severe chronic illnesses and disorders affecting the elderly in the Netherlands are chronic lung disease, heart disease, peripheral vascular disease, diabetes, strokes, joint disorders, dementia, depression and impaired hearing and vision (Deeg *et al.* 2000).

More women than men suffer from chronic illnesses in all age categories and the incidence of chronic illness increases with age (SCP 2001; Deeg *et al.* 1998, 2000). Data on chronic illness say little about the consequences this has for day-to-day functioning but data on physical impairments do so and these are fairly common among older people. Research on this subject refers to the 'geriatric giants' – the health complaints that have the strongest negative impact on the daily lives of older people (Gussekloo *et al.* 2000): mental function; mobility; stability and falling; vision and hearing; incontinence (Deeg *et al.* 1998; Deeg *et al.* 2000). Older people suffer motor limitations relatively more frequently (Deeg *et al.* 1998; Deeg *et al.* 2000) and this has an impact on their domestic activities.

General practitioners are the most frequently consulted health providers. Their knowledge of the problems facing older people is of crucial importance because, more than in other phases of life, there is a correlation between different complaints in old age. Preventing the onset of new complaints and accidents is important (SCP 2001).

Mental health

Psychological problems affect a fairly large percentage of older people. Here again, the cause often lies in the past. Predisposition (a vulnerability acquired in youth) and very negative war experiences are partially responsible for psychological problems in later life. For others problems arise due to loss experienced in later life: the loss of a partner, loss of their own health or of social contact lead relatively frequently to depression and anxiety disorders. The consequences of psychological disorders are also far reaching and often lead to cognitive and physical impairments and greatly undermine the wellbeing and social functioning of the individual (SCP 2001).

The three mental disorders most commonly affecting the older people are anxiety, depression and cognitive disability (SCP 2001) and older women

Table 4.4 Prevalence of three psychological disorders among 55–85 year olds in the Netherlands 1992/93 (%)

	Age category			Total		
	55–64 years	65–74 years	75–85 years	Men	Women	all
Anxiety*	6.9	13.9	10.4	7	13	10.2
Depression**	11.1	13.7	19	11.2	18.3	14.9
Cognitive disorders	3.4	6.1	19.3	9.5	10.9	10.2

* In a period of six months
** In a period of one week
Source: SCP (2001).

suffer more often than older men (Table 4.4). The incidence of cognitive disability and depression increases with age, while anxiety is most common among 65 to 74 year olds (SCP 2001).

Other mental health issues occur with some frequency among older people and a loss can be one of the most important psychological problems in later life (Buijssen and Polspoel 1999). At least 250,000 over 55 year olds experience loneliness as a serious problem (Linneman 1999; SCP 2001: 119). Between 40–50 per cent of older people have difficulty sleeping; half of these use sleeping aids continuously (Declerck and Verbeek 1999; SCP 2001).

The takeup of peripatetic mental healthcare (provided by the Regional Institutes for Mental Welfare (RIAGG)), is strikingly low, with only a fraction of the target group being reached. Older people with cognitive disorders present a different picture: their medical consumption is no higher than average and they have frequent contact with the RIAGG (especially those with dementia) (SCP 2001). Criticism of the help for older people with psychological problems is increasing. The consequences of psychological disorders for daily functioning and the wellbeing of older people are often so serious that help is urgently needed. The suffering and the loss of QoL resulting from common psychological disorders are unnecessary because these problems are generally easy to treat (Beekman *et al.* 1998; De Beurs *et al.* 1999; Hendriks *et al.* 1999; Penninx *et al.* 1999; Geerlings *et al.* 2000; SCP 2001). Many also observe that the psychological problems of older people are often not recognized by care workers and that the help that is given often consists only of the incorrect administering of the wrong drugs (Beekman *et al.* 1998; Nisenson *et al.* 1998; Cuijpers 1999; De Beurs *et al.* 1999; Draper 1999; Hendriks *et al.* 1999; SCP, 2001: 134).

Financial status and employment

Between 1996 and 1998 the income of older people rose a little (454 euros per year). The most important reason for this was the increase in the tax relief for this group, which has primarily benefited single older people and those with a low income. It is expected that the new tax plan will bring about a further improvement in purchasing power. In the future there will also be a group of older people who have to manage with a low income. This group consists of those who have not saved at all or have saved insufficiently for their retirement (this includes many women and minorities) and who will only receive an old age pension from the state (SCP 2001).

Single women most frequently have a low income and least often a high income. The high percentage of over-75s with a low income is reflected in this figure: the very elderly in the Netherlands are mostly women. In 1998 the proportion of single women with a low income was approximately 29 per cent and approximately 18 per cent of single men had a low income. Older couples have a low income least often, and the reduction in the number of low incomes is most notable in this group: 7 per cent had a low income in 1998 (SCP 2001).

All people aged over 65 receive the state pension and this is the most important source of income for most of them, particularly those aged over 75 (Table 4.5). Between 1990 and 1998 the supplementary pension did increase in importance, and there is a growing proportion of older people, both among the 65 to 74 year olds and among the over-75s, for whom their supplementary pension is the most important source of income. Thirty-one per cent of men receive a supplementary pension compared with 8 per cent of women. More than half those aged 65

Table 4.5 Main sources of income of people over 65 years and living independently 1998

	Age		Men	Women
	65–74 years	> 75 years	> 65 years	> 65 years
Population (× 1000)	1180	930	860	1250
with only state pension	450	330	130	650
with more than state pension	730	600	730	600

Source: SCP 2001.

or over receive more than state pension alone (largely supplementary pension) and this group increased in size in the 1990s (SCP 2001: 60–1).

Older people in residential care homes often have an extremely limited income and thus have to survive with pocket money and a clothing allowance once fixed living costs are paid (SCP 2001).

Employment in later life

The labour participation rate of older people has been in decline since 1978, as more and more older workers left the job market years before reaching statutory retirement age. In the last few years, however, this downward trend appears to have reversed. According to the SCP (2001) the proportion of men aged 50 to 64 in paid employment in 2000 was 64 per cent, and of women 31 per cent. The labour participation rate of older people is still considerably lower than that of younger adults. In all age categories many more men than women perform paid work (SCP 2001).

Unlike men, the labour participation rate of women aged 50 to 60 has steadily increased in recent decades. At present, two to three times as many women aged 50 to 55 are working as in 1973. The labour participation rate of 60-year-old women has returned to the level of 26 years earlier, but the percentage of women aged over 60 who are working is still smaller than in the early 1970s. Since 1997 the labour participation of men aged 60 and over has increased for the first time but for women in this age group remained virtually unchanged. The fact that the labour participation of 60- to 64-year-old men is now also rising suggests that the changes in early retirement schemes, which have been incorporated in most Collective Labour Agreements in recent years, are beginning to have an impact. The increase in the labour participation of 55- to 59-year-old men could largely be explained by the fact that fewer and fewer older men were becoming unemployed (SCP 2001).

A small section of the population wants to work until the official retirement age. In order to encourage people to work to this age, these individuals sometimes receive a financial bonus if they do so (Henkens 2001). Government policy is aimed at increasing the labour participation of older people with a view to making pensions more affordable. Increasing the activity rate of older people could also help to combat the labour shortages that have manifested themselves in recent years (SCP 2001: 30) and, recently, temporary agencies for people aged 65 or over have been started. More and more employers are seeing the benefits of older workers due to the fact that they contribute less social insurance for someone who is working after retirement age (Henkens 2001).

Uncertainty or dissatisfaction about the possibilities of stopping work before the official retirement age stimulates people to take out private insurance. Research shows that half of the participants in company savings accounts are using these to improve their provision for old age. More than half of the people arrange savings and annuity to be able to stop working earlier (Henkens 2001).

Early retirement

Since the 1920s the official retirement age in the Netherlands has been 65 years but working until retirement age has become an unusual phenomenon. A striking shift has taken place in the exit pattern of men since 1993–94. The two exit peaks at age 57 and age 60, which characterized the pattern in 1993–94 increased in 1998–99, to 58 and 61 years respectively. This shift indicates that the changes in early retirement schemes are starting to have an effect on the age at which people leave the labour force (SCP 2001). The percentage of men stopping work between the ages of 50–57 has fallen considerably. The most striking change in the exit pattern of women is the emergence of a peak at age 60. Although few women aged over 50 were working in 1973, those who did have paid employment often continued to work beyond their 60th birthday. By contrast, of the much larger number of women around age 50 who are currently working, the majority leave the labour force before reaching the age of 60. Continuing to work after age 60 is, however, still very rare among women (SCP 2001).

Leaving the labour market involves a major change in people's lives. It does not mean they are no longer active; some of them go on to perform unpaid voluntary work for example (see below), providing informal help (looking after their grandchildren or caring for a sick family member) and/or pursuing hobbies. Leaving the labour market is not a problem-free process for all older people, particularly where people lose their jobs unexpectedly and involuntarily, for example, due to compulsory redundancy or incapacity, in many cases this leads to a reduced feeling of wellbeing (SCP 1998, 2001) often accompanied by feelings of incompetence. Moreover, these people often face a major drop in income. Another negative aspect of leaving employment is that work-related social contacts disappear. Older people, and particularly men, will have to invest in their social network in this phase of their lives. However, retirement also offers opportunities. The fact that people have to restructure their lives to accommodate the large amount of additional free time creates the opportunity for them to opt for a healthy, active lifestyle and to build up and maintain a social network.

100

Investments of this nature can bear fruit in later life. The disappearance of employment-related obligations also offers opportunities for the government and for community organizations, which could make use of these experienced people for all manner of community tasks (SCP 2001).

Inequalities in quality of life

Gender differences

Single women most frequently have a low income, and least often a high income. In 1998 the proportion of single women with a low income was approximately 29 per cent as compared with approximately 18 per cent of single men. In all age categories more men than women perform paid work (SCP 2001). Since 1997 the labour participation of men aged 60 and over has increased but for women in this age group it has remained virtually unchanged. Different studies show that friendship is more important for older women than for older men. Women tend to have more contacts with friends in advanced years and they often use the support of friends for coping with the loss of their partner (Stevens 1998).

The older people are, the less they take part in voluntary activities. The only exception is women in the age group 55 and 59; this is probably because, as mentioned earlier, members of this age group in particular provide a great deal of informal help within their own network; and women provide this type of help more often than men. Among the over-65s, by contrast, the proportion of men is higher than that of women. It may be that these people do a lot of administrative work, an activity that is carried out mainly by men, often in later life.

More women than men suffer from chronic illnesses, anxiety, depression and cognitive disorders. Women mention more often unfavourable health conditions, they experience their health more often as 'moderate' or 'bad' and make more use of care services.

Age differences

The over-75s more often have a lower income than younger older people. Despite the increase in recent years, the labour participation rate of older people is still considerably lower than that of younger adults. Whereas more than three out of four people aged 35 to 49 perform paid work, this applies for only two out of three persons aged 50 to 54, half those aged 55 to 59 and only one in seven of 60 to 64 year olds. There are virtually no (paid) workers among the over-65s and only one in 40 people aged 65 to 74 are still in paid employment.

Older people are more content than younger people with their residential setting in general and experience less nuisance from odour, dust, noise or traffic. This pattern of a satisfaction level that increases with age also occurs within the older population: the over-75s have fewer problems with their residential setting than the 'younger old'.

More than half the 'young old' (65 to 74 years) and almost two-thirds of the very elderly have one or more chronic disorders. The incidence of chronic illness increases with age. The incidence of cognitive disorders and depression increases with age, while anxiety is most common among 65 to 74 year olds.

People in the older age categories assess their health as poor more often than younger people, but from the age of 75 onwards there is little further increase in the feeling of being unwell: slightly less than a fifth of the very old feel not very healthy. The Leiden-85+ study showed that 75 per cent of the very elderly living at home who were questioned, all aged 85 or more, assessed their health as 'good' to 'very good' (Gussekloo *et al.* 2000). Residents of sheltered housing or institutions assessed their own health more negatively than those living independently. These differences disappear for people aged 85 and over; this group assessed its own health as poor or moderate roughly just as often.

The membership rate of associations or community organizations decreases with age; 74 per cent of those aged under 75 are members, compared with 50 per cent of over-75s. The biggest difference between older people and younger people occurs with sports associations, where 'young people' are roughly 4.5 times more likely to be members than older people. People in the 55 to 74 age group are more often members of a hobby, choral, music or amateur dramatic society than people aged under 55 or over 75. A distinction can be drawn within the organizations concerned mainly with furthering a certain interest (such as a political party or an organization with a community object) and associations that are of a more social nature (such as sports or hobby associations). Membership rates decline with increasing age in both types of association, though this is most marked in social clubs.

In general, the older people are the less voluntary work they do. Those aged 50 to 64 perform voluntary work slightly less frequently (approximately 62 per cent) than 35 to 49 year olds (66 per cent). After age 65 participation in voluntary work declines, and is especially low among the over-75s (26 per cent). As regards the number of voluntary activities a person carries out, it is striking that, compared with 50 to 59 year olds, 60 to 64 year olds relatively frequently perform several activities. In other words, those people who do voluntary work are more often active on several fronts. Roughly one-third of those aged under

75 provide informal help within their own network. Those aged 55 to 59 give informal help slightly more often than the other age groups; it may be that this group more often has a combination of small grandchildren and needy parents.

People more often feel lonely or downcast as they grow older. By contrast, older people less frequently feel out of sorts or restless than people aged under 55. Over 20 per cent of the over-75s suffer frequently or very frequently from feeling lonely or downcast – roughly twice as many as people aged 35 to 54. After adjusting for the other factors, age does not affect wellbeing. In other words, the previously noted differences between people in various age categories are to a large extent caused by the fact that very elderly people suffer more frequently from health problems and more frequently live alone.

Variations in income and economic situation

The higher their socio-economic status, the more time older people spend outside their home and the more diverse their pattern of activities. Personal computer ownership turns out to depend partly on income, education level, household composition and gender. These differences can also be observed within age categories; older people with a high income and high education level have a PC at home much more often than their less well off and less well educated peers.

Socio-economic circumstances are mainly of indirect significance for loneliness. Those with a higher education and a higher income have in general larger networks and are therefore less vulnerable to loneliness (Dykstra and Gierveld 1999).

Ethnic minority older people

There are currently more than 90,000 over-55s of ethnic (non-Western) origin in the Netherlands, of whom about 40,000 are Turkish and Moroccan and over 33,000 are Surinamese or Antillean. By far the majority of them will grow older in the Netherlands. The number of older people from ethnic minorities will therefore greatly increase in the future (SCP 2001: 310).

Elderly Turks and Moroccans have barely integrated into Dutch society while the integration of older Surinamese and Antilleans is much further advanced. The economic, social and cultural gap between older Turks and Moroccans and the indigenous society is extremely wide. Their health is also poorer than that of older persons from the other groups investigated. Many older Turks and Moroccans are on the margins of Dutch society. Their level of inactivity is high and many have very low incomes, on which they say they can get by barely if at all. From time to time older Turks and Moroccans who are no longer economically active make calls for labour force participation to be promoted, but many of them have little or no education, are virtually illiterate and have little knowledge of Dutch. Many have also been out of the labour market for some time. Persuading employers to take them on, as well as encouraging older Turks and Moroccans to focus on the labour market, will not be straightforward.

The position of older Surinamese and Antilleans differs radically from those of older Turks and Moroccans. In various respects they barely differ from indigenous older persons. They have managed to secure a reasonably good socio-economic position and are also well integrated in social and cultural terms. Among other things this may be attributed to the migration history of these groups. A substantial proportion of the older Surinamese and Antilleans came from the upper strata of (former) Surinamese and Antillean society. In particular, they have used education as a way to integrate in the Netherlands. This picture does not apply to all older Surinamese and Antilleans: those with less education and who often came as labour immigrants or at an early age with their family have not managed to carve out such a favourable position. All things considered, however, a good many older Surinamese and Antilleans can be considered to have integrated successfully, which cannot be said of the older Turks and Moroccans (SCP 2001: 280–1).

Conclusion

The Netherlands is moving from a relatively young population in the European context towards a relatively old one. The Dutch government is fully aware of this shift and has made preparations to cope with its consequences in many areas, sometimes successful, sometimes less so. The Netherlands also has a long tradition of measuring the QoL of its citizens.

Note

1. The NESTOR study was a national cross-sectional study conducted in 1992 among people aged 55–85 (n = 4500), which focussed on social networks and lifecourse data. The Longitudinal Ageing Study Amsterdam (LASA) built on NESTOR with a longitudinal study of the social, cognitive, emotional and physical dimensions of ageing. The fourth round of observation was undertaken in 2002. (Deeg and Westendorp-de Seriere 1994; Deeg *et al.* 1998; http://www.ssg.scw.vu.nl/lasa)

Sweden: quality of life in old age I

Lars Andersson

Definition and measurement of quality of life

Social reporting was initiated in Sweden in the early 1970s. Since 1974 Statistics Sweden has conducted annual interview studies (ULF) with national representative samples of the population aged 16 to 84 (initially up to the age of 74). Due to the upper age limit of 84 years, less is known about the 200,000 older people (mostly women living alone) who are over 85 years of age.

Measurements are mainly based on 'objective' indicators in that the initiators of the study wanted to avoid any possible scepticism that could result from a public authority publishing subjective opinions expressed by the population. They also wanted to avoid the problem of 'false awareness'. Consequently the term 'living conditions' was used instead of the term 'quality of life' (QoL). The living conditions comprised ten social domains: education, employment, working environment, finances, housing conditions, transport and communication, recreation, social relations, political participation, and health. Later the indicators also covered social mobility and violence. Much of the data in this chapter and Chapter 10 originate from the ULF studies.

As in the case of the chapters on the Netherlands, this chapter makes use of Veenhoven's (2000) conceptualization of QoL, which distinguishes between opportunities for a good life (life chances) and the good life itself (life results) – the difference between potentiality and actuality. She also makes a distinction between outer qualities and inner qualities. The four are combined in a matrix, with the concepts liveability, life-ability, utility of life, and appreciation of life. The term 'life' in this instance is used not only for the aggregate older people, but also for individual older people.

The publications used in this review of QoL in old age in Sweden are listed in the four quadrants in Table 5.1. According to Veenhoven, the quadrant 'utility of life' represents the notion that a good life must be good for something more than itself, that is it presumes some higher values.

In 1989, Tornstam introduced his gerotranscendence theory. This is described as a shift in metaperspective from a materialistic and rational view to a more cosmic and transcendent one, normally followed by an increase in life satisfaction. The development of gerotranscendence is seen as a 'natural' process that has been obstructed by the structures of modern Western societies. Tornstam (1997) has found patterns of increasing cosmic transcendence, coherence, and need for solitude. The theory has gained some influence in Scandinavia, especially in nursing science, but lately it has been criticized for being empirically weak, and having parallels in the New Age movement as well as in romantic orientalism (Jönson and Magnusson 2001).

Torres (1999, 2001), working with the concept of successful ageing, sets out to shed light on how the process of migration to a culture that significantly differs from one's culture of origin can challenge the manner in which successful ageing is understood. She formulates a culturally relevant theoretical framework for the study of notions of successful ageing. She reaches the conclusion that not only are understandings of successful ageing contextually determined, they are also much more processual than has been assumed.

Table 5.1 Publications used in this review

	Outer qualities	**Inner qualities**
	Liveability	**Life-ability**
Life chances	Trydegård (2000)	Öberg (1997)
	Johansson (1997)	Trossholmen (2000)
	Andersson (1999)	Persson *et al.* (2001)
	Winqvist (1999)	
	Andersson (2002)	
	Jönson (2001)	
	Utility of life	**Appreciation of life**
Life results	Tornstam (1989)	Hillerås (2001)
	Torres (2001)	

Environments of ageing

Housing is a very important aspect of the QoL of older people. Obviously they spend much more time at home than individuals from other age categories. Large-scale time-use studies are scarce in Sweden and most data are outdated. However, time use is not subject to dramatic changes. A general observation is that a large part of the day is spent at home – for older people in Sweden about 80 to 85 per cent, that is 20 out of the 24 hours (Andersson 1988).

Generally, people aged 55 and over do not move house as often as other age groups. When people do move, two main directions have been identified – one to the city centre and another to districts with a particular nature or cherished cultural values. City centres in Sweden are attractive due to their lack of inner city slums. Thus an empty-nest couple may sell their house and move to an apartment in the city centre, but this is only true for Stockholm (SOU 2002: 29). Another direction is to spend much more time at one's summer home. In contrast to other Nordic countries, such as Norway and Finland, permanent or temporary migration to southern Europe has not been studied much in Sweden.

Housing for older people does not differ from the housing of the general population in any major respect (except when the question of institutionalization arises). However, since people do not move so frequently, certain generations dominate in areas and types of buildings that were in fashion when they became settled. In the 65 to 74 age group, 57 per cent live in houses and 42 per cent in apartments. In the 75 to 84 age group the corresponding numbers are 41 per cent and 51 per cent. In both age groups about 4 per cent live in cramped conditions – the definition being that they have less than one bedroom per person (a couple cohabiting is assumed to share a bedroom), kitchen and living room not included. One exception to the regular housing is the senior housing, of which there were 11,000 apartments in 1999. Usually, it is necessary to be 55 and over to move there, and the housing is based on some kind of community (SOU 2002: 29).

Research on the quality of housing shows that the major obstructions to accessibility in apartments are lack of handles next to the WC and the bath, and that the cupboard under the kitchen sink may not be reachable. It is possible to apply to the municipality for a home adaptation grant to solve these inconveniences. In 1999 more than 55,000 such grants were made. However, generally, the main obstacle to accessibility is the lack of lifts. Unfortunately the statistics on lifts are inadequate. Statistics Sweden gives data on the number of households on the third floor and higher that do not have access to lifts. Thus, nothing is known about the situation for those on the first and second floors, and if it is necessary to use stairs to be able to get out despite the presence of the lift. According to the available data about 12 per cent to 13 per cent of households in the age group 45 and over who live in apartments do not have access to an lift. The only exception is the age group 80 and over in rented apartments, where only 5 per cent lack lifts (Table 5.2). This is probably because of movement to institutions (SOU 2002: 29).

Table 5.2 Access to lifts in rented apartments 1999 (%)

	Age of tenant					
	45–59	60–4	65–9	70–4	75–9	80+
1–2nd floor	68	64	71	64	67	68
3rd floor						
– lift	8	7	6	7	7	11
– no lift	10	10	7	11	9	5
4th+ floor						
– lift	12	15	15	16	16	15
– no lift	2	3	0	2	0	0

Source: SOU (2002: 29).

According to a survey reported in SOU (2002: 29), four out of ten people aged 55 to 64 had to use stairs to enter and leave the place where they live (in spite of a lift, if any), and six out of ten had stairs inside.

The survey also included questions about wishes and planning for housing in old age. Nine out of ten considered closeness to public transport and in-house services important. The same holds true for closeness to nature and the presence of a balcony or terrace. Eight out of ten consider it important to receive help with cleaning, shopping and so on, and to live with people in all age groups. Less important is closeness to entertainment or to live with age peers. Many consider the latter to be the least important. On the other hand, three out of four had made no decision about housing in old age, and one out of three had not thought about it at all (SOU 2002: 29).

New technology

In 2000 about 20 per cent in the age group 65 to 84 had access to a computer at home (28 per cent aged 65 to 74, and 11 per cent aged 75 to 84). In the age group 16 to 64, three out of four had access to a computer at home. The figures for access to the Internet at home are of course lower (17 per cent among those aged 65 to 74, and 5 per cent among those aged 75 to 84). The figure for the age group 16 to 64 is 63 per cent. The differences between the groups are slowly decreasing as the growth rates in the use of computers and of the Internet are almost inversely correlated with the level of usage just a few years earlier (SOU 2002: 15).

The use of modern technology for caring and other purposes has been tried in various projects in Sweden. One of these is ACTION (Assisting Carers using Telematics Interventions to meet Older Persons' Needs), which is funded by the European Commission (Magnusson *et al.* 2001). Participating countries, in addition to Sweden, are Ireland, Portugal and the UK. The aim of the project is to support disabled and frail older people and their family carers, to enhance or maintain their autonomy, independence and QoL by providing comprehensive information, advice and support in their daily life.

The majority of the Swedish carers (n = 40) voiced enthusiastic expectations in relation to the ACTION services, and had their homes adapted in order to become connected to the health and social services (n = 13). Thus the carers saw ACTION as potentially being able to provide information and support that was not currently provided by formal health and social service providers. One explanation for the interest in the project is probably to be found in the rapid uptake of information and communication technology within Swedish society as a whole. Thus, the majority of the Swedish carers displayed a high level of receptivity to ACTION. This supports findings by Zimmer and Chappell (1999) who concluded that new technology that focused on enhancing the QoL for older people in their homes would be welcomed by many.

ACTION's multimedia programmes have been evaluated by the majority of users as helpful, easy to use and understand, as well as useful and informative. The videophone has been used for consultations between family carers and the local health and social service professionals with practical benefits in terms of information giving, education and support. A practical benefit of the telematic interventions is that they are designed to reduce feelings of isolation for those family carers who are geographically distant from the health and care centres or live far away from their relatives, or cannot practically leave their homes.

Transport

To be able to live a normal life in the community the opportunity to travel is essential. If older people are to participate in different activities then the transportation system must be adapted to their needs and special requisites for mobility. One way to do this is to use service routes. A service route is a bus service that is an integrated part of the regular public transport system but has been specially adapted for people with diminished mobility. The idea behind service routes is to provide older and handicapped people with the possibility of using public transportation more often and more spontaneously by deliberately decreasing walking distances, facilitating getting on and off, and lowering the risk for accidents. Accordingly, it will be easier to do shopping on one's own and it will increase the opportunity for meeting others and strengthening social networks, that is to enhance the QoL.

The first service routes in Stockholm started in 1988 on a trial basis. The service became permanent in 1989. Presently there are 23 service routes in the county of Stockholm, of which ten are run in the city of Stockholm. The service routes are administered by the Regional Transport Company (SL). The main aim of the programme is to make travelling available for everyone. The objectives are to (a) adapt public transport to the disabled, (b) counteract the rising expenses for the Special Transportation Services (STS), and (c) offer a means whereby the transport companies can make adjustments to the market and inform the public about the availability of services.

Sweden, like many other EU countries, offered STS as an initial approach for solving the transportation problems of older people and the disabled. In 1990, 5 per cent of the total population in Sweden was entitled to use the service. The expenditure for STS amounts to about 15 per cent of the total costs for public transportation services. However, there is still a large group of people who cannot use conventional public transportation but are not so seriously disabled that they are eligible for the comprehensive service offered by STS.

The main target groups for service routes are all older and disabled people who have difficulties in using, or have no access to, ordinary public transport. However, the service routes are available to anyone who wants to use them. In order to implement a service route at least 1000 older people must live within 200 metres of the proposed route. The route layout makes walking distances shorter. The buses run between approximately 9 am and 3 pm. There is one bus per route. The routes are operated by small buses featuring low boarding steps, wheelchair ramps, extra handles and railings inside. The driving time is adjusted so that the driver can help the passengers on and off the bus. The driver gains experience and familiarity with the passengers.

In general, it can be said that service route operating costs are higher per vehicle-kilometre and per vehicle-hour than those for other bus services, since this service has a lower average velocity. On the other hand, several service routes have enjoyed higher occupancy than that of bus services on average. The service routes have been assessed using outcome evaluations, including economic evaluation. Moreover, as a part of the Mégapoles project, the service routes in Stockholm have been evaluated using a peer review tool (Andersson 1999).

The Swedish Transport Research Board found that between 40 and 50 per cent of all people over 65 encounter several types of problems on ordinary bus trips. For example, they have difficulties in getting to the bus stop and when getting on or off the bus. On service routes, the number of people who have problems has been shown to be less than 10 per cent. The report from the Swedish Transport Research Board concluded that service routes are good for municipalities because they seem to put the brakes on rising expenses for STS. It has also been speculated whether service routes would be good for county councils, which could reduce the pressure on care facilities. Disabled and older people could gain greater mobility and be able to live at home longer. These types of cross-sector benefits are difficult to calculate although some attempts have been made (Fowkes *et al.* 1994).

The SL counts the number of passengers on the service routes twice a year. They also interview users, using both fixed and open-ended response alternatives. About half of the passengers are in the age span 70 to 79 years of age, and about 20 per cent between 80 and 89 years of age. It has been shown that about 20 per cent of the passengers would have either refrained from travelling or would have to use the STS if there were no service route. Thus, for the older people, service routes have brought about greater personal mobility and less dependence on other people and institutions. They are also experienced as a new and stimulating opportunity to make contact with other people.

Transport is not the first thing that comes to mind when social networks and QoL are discussed. Optimal public transport, however, may be an efficient tool for giving older people the opportunity to keep up social contacts and to remain integrated in society. Service routes have been shown to be an important influence on social contacts among older people.

Physical and mental health

In December 2003 the population of Sweden was approximately 8.98 million, of which 17.2 per cent was 65 years of age and over. The proportion of people aged 80 and above was 5.3 per cent. The life expectancy for a newly born girl was 82.43 years and for a boy 77.91 years. The number of persons in the age group 65 and over is expected to increase by 25 per cent over the coming two decades.

Good health has long been considered a very important, if not the most important, condition for a high QoL. When people are asked about the most important prerequisite for a good life, the answer in most cases is to remain healthy. However, if struck by a health problem, it is common for them to cope with the new situation and argue that they have learned to enjoy life (perhaps even more) despite the disease or the injury. This adaptation can be called 'selective optimization with compensation' (Baltes and Baltes 1990).

The health data presented here are largely based upon the annual Statistics Sweden Surveys of Living Conditions (Persson *et al.* 2001; Statistics Sweden 2000). These surveys cover ages up to 85 (see above), and the description is in most cases limited to the 65 to 84 year age group. Overall, the self-reported health in this age group has improved during the 20 years since the mid-1980s, although the picture is ambiguous. The proportion who regard their health as poor has declined. For example, mobility has improved and the proportion of disabilities has decreased, as has the proportion of ADL difficulties. Vision has improved but hearing has deteriorated in some groups.

Thus, perceived health has improved among older people but there is no corresponding reduction in the prevalence of long-term illness. Rather, a tendency to an increase can be discerned among women aged 65 to 74 and among men aged 75 to 84. Moreover, more older people were receiving medical treatment for their long-term illnesses in 2004 than in the mid-1980s. Of the long-term diseases reported, those of the circulatory organs predominated. Close to half of all women and men aged 75 to 84 have some sort of circulatory problems. Heart diseases are three to five times more common among retired people than in the population as a whole. A report from the Stockholm Gerontology Research Center in 1997 (Styrborn 1997) showed that about 80 per cent of people over 77 had two or more chronic conditions, while about 8 per cent were in full health, with or without problems of vision and hearing.

Some types of pain decrease after retirement, which may be due to a fall in physical activity. Such a tendency exists, for example, for backache, particularly among men. Women report pain to a greater extent than men. The prevalence of pain decreased during the 1980s for both men and women but increased during the 1990s. However, severe pain decreased during the 1990s (for 65 to 74 year olds).

A little less than one-third of the 65- to 74-year-old men and a little more than half of those aged 75 to 84 judged themselves unable to run a short distance (approximately 100 metres). For women, the percentage points are 10 per cent higher. Disability, measured as the inability to get on a bus without difficulty or to take a fairly short walk at a reasonably fast pace, has decreased by one-third among 65 to 74 year olds and by two-thirds among 75 to 84 year olds, since the mid-1970s. An increased level of hip and knee joint surgery may partly explain this change. Mobility has improved in all socio-economic groups and for both sexes, but mobility problems are more common among former blue-collar workers.

Impaired vision, defined as the inability to read normal text in a daily news-paper with or without glasses, afflicts somewhat more than 3 per cent of 65 to 74 year olds and about 8 per cent of 75 to 84 year olds. Vision has improved since the end of the 1980s, particularly among women who have had white-collar occupations. This improvement may be explained by an increasing amount of cataract surgery. Impaired hearing is most common among former blue-collar men, among whom about 40 per cent are affected – a figure that has increased since 1990. Among former white-collar workers a little less than 28 per cent have impaired hearing, a figure that has decreased during the same period. According to the H-70 study, just over half of 70 year olds were toothless in 1971. Five years later the proportion was 38 per cent, in 1981 it was 35 per cent and in 1992 it was down to 17 per cent. The proportion of older people who do not take any physical exercise appears unchanged since the end of the 1980s, while the proportion who take regular exercise appears to have increased. Approximately a fifth of men and just over a quarter of women take no exercise.

The prevalence of osteoporosis has increased sharply during the past few years – 7 per cent of 50- to 59-year-old women have osteoporosis, 22 per cent aged 60 to 69, 31 per cent aged 70 to 79 and 36 per cent aged 80 to 89. The pro-portion of older people over 75 hospitalized by fractures has increased since 1987. Hip fractures are the most common type of fracture and occur twice as often in women as in men. Hip fractures have increased by 15 per cent among men since 1987 but have been relatively unchanged among women. Lower arm fractures have increased particularly among women, while vertebral fractures have increased somewhat more among men.

Two major longitudinal studies in Sweden – the H-70 study in Göteborg and the Kungsholmen study in Stockholm – show that mental disorders increase with age. In the former study, one in four 70 year olds and a third of

79 year olds had serious mental disturbances, including dementia, and in the latter study 15 per cent of the 75 year olds had mental disorders. The H-70 study showed that three-quarters of those who committed suicide had had some form of anti-depressive treatment. The Kungsholmen study showed that over half of those with death wishes also had psychiatric diagnoses (Forsell 2000a). Suicide has declined in men over 75 years, although the frequency is still just over 1.5 times as high as among men in general and five times as common as among women of corresponding ages. Using Kungsholmen data, Forsell (2000b) has also examined predictors for depression, anxiety and psychotic symptoms in a population with a mean age of 84.5 years. Having started with several indicators of socio-demographic variables, use of care, somatic and psychiatric variables, disabilities and social network, it eventually turned out that depression, anxiety and, in part, psychotic symptoms mostly affect people who had been affected earlier in life. Thus these problems in very old people are linked to a lifetime psychological vulnerability.

It is disputed whether extended life expectancy involves more 'healthy' years or more years with disease and pain. The Statistics Sweden Health Index, a measure combining mortality and morbidity, shows that only part of the additional years are free from disease. Between the mid-1980s and 2004 there were 0.2 more years with full health for both sexes between the ages 65 to 84. The number of years with somewhat impaired health increased by 2.1 years for men and 1.6 years for women in the same age group.

Income and employment

The national pension scheme includes a basic pension (folkpension) and a supplementary pension (ATP). The ATP is based on income from gainful employment whereas the right to a basic pension is based on residence in Sweden. Effective from 1999, a new pension system is gradually replacing the basic pension and ATP. In addition to the new scheme, most people qualify for contractual pensions/occupational pensions and may also have personal pension savings.

The economic situation of older people improved during the 1990s. While the median income for the whole population (24 to 84 years) increased by 5 per cent from 1989/90 to 1997, it increased by 10 per cent in the 65 to 74 age group and by 34 per cent in the 75 to 84 age group. In 1999, 1.5 per cent of the pensioners in Sweden were on social assistance. People born abroad made up nearly 60 per cent of those on social assistance, mainly because they were in most cases not entitled to full basic retirement pension.

The average income of pensioners improved relative to the rest of the population during the 1990s because new cohorts of pensioners with higher pensions have replaced older cohorts of pensioners with lower pensions, and the economic crises in the early part of the 1990s affected the adult cohorts to a higher degree. Defining low incomes as 50 per cent of the median income of all individuals, the proportion of pensioners with such a low income has been around 1 per cent during the last decade, while the percentage in the rest of the population has been 4 to 5 per cent. With regard to disposable income (income from work, capital, and transfers, after tax) women aged 66 to 72, 73 to 79 and 80 and over have about the same income as men in the oldest age group. While the income for men in the two younger age groups has decreased somewhat during the 1990s, it is still more than 25 per cent higher than that of women in the same age groups.

The oldest generations possess lower net capital than those who are middle-aged. However, from 1994 to 2004 the proportion of the total net capital possessed by the oldest generations has increased. This could mean that, in the future, intergenerational gifts and inheritance will become even more important than today (Table 5.3).

Net capital in most cases is made up of the value of the dwelling. Figure 5.1 shows the size of the financial assets in addition to the net capital in six age groups in 1999. Although the oldest pensioners possess a lower net capital, the difference in financial assets is fairly small.

In total, the sources of income for pensioners are made up of pensions (87 per cent), income from capital (9 per cent), and work (4 per cent), while other sources of income amounted to less than 1 per cent.

Table 5.3 Total net capital of households (%)

Age of 'Head of household'	1992	1993	1997	1999
	Percentage of net property			
25–44	20.4	16.4	17.9	15.4
45–64	46.3	44.8	46.0	46.2
65+	32.1	36.4	34.7	37.1

Source: SOU (2002: 29).

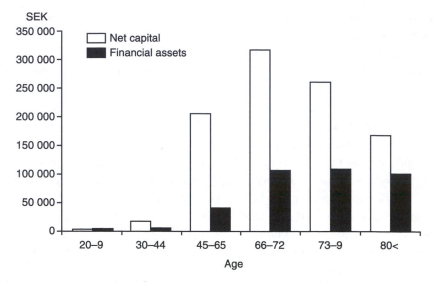

Figure 5.1 Net capital and financial assets in 1999 (median SEK)
Source: Ds 2002: 14

With regard to material circumstances, the Eurobarometer of 1992 included a question on the ownership of consumer durables in the household (Andersson 1993; Walker 1993). The list contained a colour TV, video recorder, video camera, radio clock, PC/home computer, still camera, electric drill, electric deep-fat fryer, two or more cars, and a second home or a holiday home/flat. A rating of the countries according to the percentage who possessed the various items revealed the following positions for older people in Sweden: 1, 2, 2, 2, 3, 1, 1, 13 (and last, for an electric deep fat fryer – luckily, from a public health perspective), 6, and 1. The general picture is one of ample material assets, in particular as the household size is small in Sweden. There is, for example, no son or daughter in the household with whom an older person shares a car.

Retirement

Retirement as a social institution has occupied a central position within gerontology from its very beginning. At the end of the 1940s old age in Sweden was a category with few models, and within the framework of the medical model it was defined in terms of misery and loss of capacities. Through the institutionalization of retirement via state pensions an acceptable pension level started to be reached after the Second World War. As noted by Jönson (2001), there was a

116

concern that the feeling of void characterizing life in old age homes would also affect a growing number of retirees.

Retirement was initially viewed with some hostility. It was seen as causing problems. Gerontologists spoke about the 'retirement shock'. In order to avoid death from retiring, it was believed that people should continue to work, or at least indulge themselves in meaningful leisure activities, or as a last resort be the target of therapeutic activities. It was argued that preferably older people should try to get a job in the open market. If that is impossible, the company doctor or the GP should try to organize occupational therapy in special institutions with more or less meaningless jobs, all in order to counteract the risk of inactivity among the older people (Jönson 2001).

With the deinstitutionalization of the lifecourse, the centrality of retirement in late-life identity has been questioned and an insecurity regarding exit from work has emerged. Today, the real retirement age is lower than the formal retirement age and although a comparatively larger proportion of the population in Sweden (compared to the rest of EU) remains in the workforce at higher ages (80 per cent at the age of 55, and 62 per cent at the age of 60), this has led to a lot of concern particularly among politicians and economists. The well known dilemma is how a decreasing number of people in the workforce and an increasing number of retirees will affect the economy.

The calculations of future pensions for the cohorts that will receive their pension within the coming decades show that the pension will be lower than expected. One solution that has been accepted in Sweden is to make it possible to continue to work from age 65 to age 67 – which was the retirement age up to 1976. This can be an excellent alternative for some people but what about the health situation in the years around retirement? Walker (1999) notes that health status has a critical bearing on the future of both pensions and retirement. The deterioration of health with age has several determinants, one of which is work life.

A report from Statistics Sweden, based on data from the ULF study, clearly shows a 'retirement levelling' or even a 'retirement dip' (that is a long lasting improvement in health) with regard to some indicators of subjective health (Statistics Sweden 2000; Andersson 2002). In a report to the parliamentary working committee 'Senior 2005', Andersson (2002) has taken a closer look at health around retirement by adding more health variables and also introducing a control for the time of retirement. A division was made between age up to 65 and years after retirement. There is also a statistical control for the effect of marital status, region, gender (where relevant) and professional category (where relevant). The new data set is based on 18,134 individuals, aged 45 to 84, interviewed during the periods 1988–89 and 1994–97. It should be emphasized that the ULF study is not a study about retirement. It is a general study of living conditions where retirement is one factor considered.

As an example of what can happen around retirement, Figure 5.2 illustrates the levelling of long-term illness in connection with retirement.

It is obvious that if the trend from the age groups 45 to 54 and 55 to 59 would have continued in the same direction, the picture would have looked quite different. Particularly for white-collar workers, it is not until five years

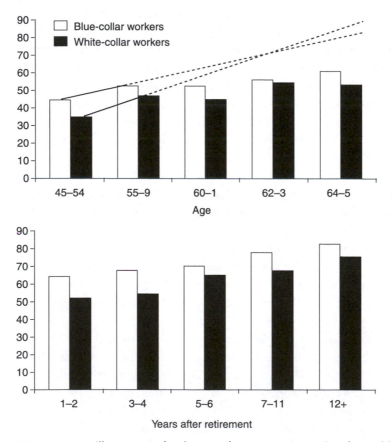

Figure 5.2 Long-term illness around retirement (percentage reporting the problem)

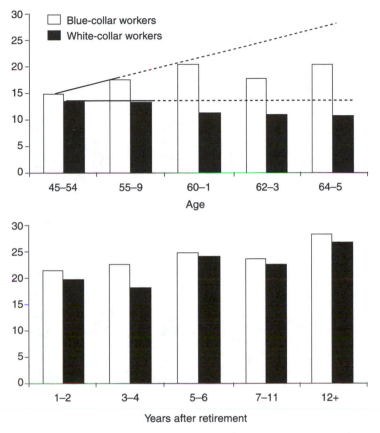

Figure 5.3 Sleep disturbances around retirement (percentage reporting the problem)

after retirement that the proportion of people reporting long-term illness increases again.

With regard to work life issues, one can identify three pathways. The first could be called 'catch up', where the health status among blue-collar workers after retirement approaches the level of white-collar workers (such as sleep disturbances – see Figure 5.3).

The second pathway is 'business as usual', where the differences between the groups remain the same after retirement. This is exemplified by general health status (Figure 5.4).

The third pathway 'delayed effects' is exemplified by physical disability, where differences between the groups show up long after retirement (Figure 5.5).

119

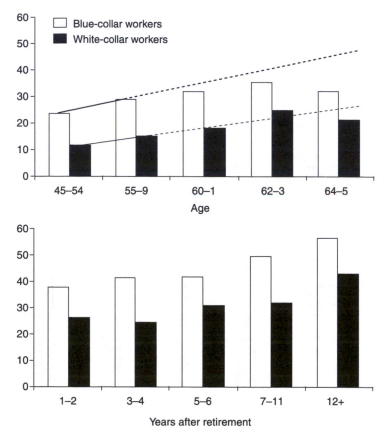

Figure 5.4 General health status around retirement (percentage reporting problem)

A final example is the figures for fatigue, which show a U-shaped curve for both men and women. It seems as if the number of people who suffer from fatigue is never as low as just around retirement age (Figure 5.6).

A challenging question is how the ambitions of the governments in many countries in the EU and elsewhere to raise the retirement age in order to secure pension systems can square with the improvement in health in connection with retirement. The observed improved health of new cohorts of older people is constantly taken as an excuse for proposals for a higher retirement age. A thought-provoking question is to what extent the improved health could be the result of people retiring as early as they do today?

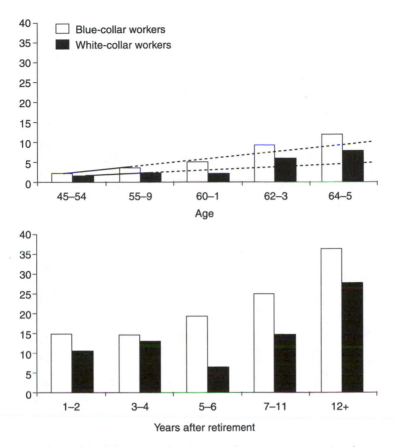

Figure 5.5 Physical disability around retirement (percentage reporting the problem)

Early retirement

Health aside, what are the attitudes of people who will retire within a decade or two? In a report from the National Institute for Working Life in Sweden, Torgén *et al.* (2001) found that about half of the respondents aged 45 to 64 were fairly certain that they would continue to work up until 65 (men 54 per cent, women 50 per cent). It should be noted, though, that in this age group about 30 per cent had already left the workforce. Considering that the respondents were a selected group the figures must be regarded as low (Table 5.4).

The answers to another question underline the low interest in continued work. Thirty-four per cent of men and 31 per cent of women claim that they

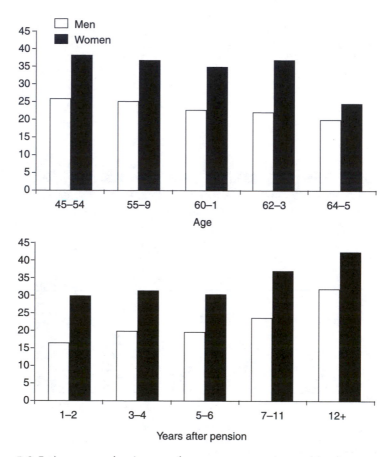

Figure 5.6 Fatigue around retirement (percentage reporting problem)

add to their savings in order to be able to stop working before retirement age if they want to. Only 13 per cent of the men and 9 per cent among women say that they hope to be able to work after retirement age in order to get a higher pension. To continue work after retirement age for intrinsic reasons – because the work is stimulating – only appeals to 15 per cent of men and 8 per cent of women.

It is notable that only about half of those still in the workforce want to continue to work until age 65, and that about three out of four say that they hope they do not have to work after retirement age. The first reason that comes to

Table 5.4 Percentage of people aged 50–64 who believe they will work until their official retirement age

Age	Men	Women
50–4	59	51
55–9	57	44
60–4	69	53

Source: SOU (2002: 29).

mind is the stressful work situation. However, it is also quite possible that the new positive image of the 'young olds' is tempting, promising a permissive life where one is economically secure and does what one wants. Thus, there is reason to believe that the economic incentive has to be quite strong in order to convince people to postpone retirement, although they are very well aware of the possible economic necessity of continued work.

The significance of age for middle-aged employees

Job advertisements may be of significance when it comes to influencing people's attitudes towards middle-aged people, and they may contribute in an indirect way to the formation of stereotypes and consequently influence people's QoL. In most Western countries, employers are reluctant to employ people over 50 years of age and sometimes even people as young as just over 40 years of age. Coexistent with this is a demographic trend characterized by a growing number of older people. In Sweden, 31 per cent of the workforce was 50 years and older in 1993, and the proportion is estimated to be 37 per cent by 2010.

Johansson (1997) tried to find out how middle-aged people look upon the significance of age in working life. Her main study is based on interviews with 24 people aged 45 to 54 years – half of them men, half of them women. She also made complementary studies regarding age in job advertisements. According to the perceptions of the respondents, age is of significance as a hindrance primarily in the recruitment process. Employers' preference for younger applicants has been explained as being due to rapid changes taking place in society, new technology and younger people's more current education. However, according to the respondents, there may be other more latent reasons as well, such as a need for sorting and categorizing people, power and control, prejudices, stereotypes, and ageism.

In total 6099 jobs advertised in the Swedish daily newspaper *Dagens Nyheter* were studied in 1992 and 1995. The frequency of specific age requirements, the most common ages mentioned and the mode of expressing age – that is verbally or by chronological age – were studied. The frequency of a specific age requirement in job advertisements was as low as 12 per cent in 1992 and 13 per cent in 1995. In addition, most of the advertisements with a specific age requirement were for salesmen, and all of the jobs, apart from eight, were associated with the private sector. Thus, the respondents' perception that most advertisements had a specific age requirement was not confirmed by the data. The most common way of expressing age was by using age intervals, and the most common age interval was 25 to 35 years.

In the *Berliner Morgenpost*, in Germany, the frequency of a specific age requirement was slightly higher, 17 per cent. In both newspapers, the use of age intervals was the most common way of expressing age. However, in the *Berliner Morgenpost* the age intervals 25 to 40 years, 30 to 40 years and 30 to 45 years were just as common as the interval 25 to 35 years. In both newspapers, ages above 45 years were very seldom in demand. Job advertisements have various functions – not only to inform job applicants – and therefore they are also read by managers and other people. Hence, as an image-producing force their influence cannot be disregarded.

Inequalities in quality of life

Inequalities have, in gerontological research in Sweden, mainly been studied in connection with health. Mortality among old people declined sharply in the 1980s and 1990s, which led to increased life expectancy. Socio-economic differences in mortality remain, at least until the age of 90, but are less pronounced than among the gainfully employed. Among men, excess mortality is approximately 25 per cent higher among those aged 65 to 84 and living alone than among those co-habiting. There is no difference for women.

In a report (Folkhälsorapport 2001) based on register data (official records) on both municipal, county and national levels various types of inequalities were highlighted (the data in most cases had an upper age limit of 84). Both average length of life and cause of death differ between housing areas with different socio-economic characteristics. In 1993–97, remaining average length of life for men aged 65 was 5.7 years longer in areas with the highest mean income compared with the areas with the lowest mean income. For women the difference was 5.2 years. The differences had increased from the years

1981–85. For men, the remaining average length of life in the wealthiest areas increased 2.1 years in this period, whereas the increase in the poorest areas was 0.7 years.

With regard to morbidity, the register data show that among married men born in Sweden, and belonging to the lowest income quintile, severe ill health is four times as common as among men in the highest income quintile. Among women severe ill health is three times as common as among those in the highest income quintile. For example, among men aged 65 to 69 the proportion with severe ill health is 12 per cent in the lowest income group, and 3 per cent in the highest group. For women, the corresponding figures are 13 and 4 per cent. Another way of looking at this difference is to conclude that the proportion of men aged 80 to 84 in the highest income quintile with severe ill health is lower than for men aged 65 to 69 in the lowest income quintile – 7 per cent and 12 per cent respectively. The same is true for women. One way of expressing this is that there is more than 15 years of health difference between the highest income group and the lowest one.

According to Statistics Sweden's Health Index, the probability of experiencing severe ill health is highest for those aged 80 to 84, single, born abroad, and having an income in the lowest income quintile. The proportion with severe ill health in this group is 36 per cent among men and 42 per cent among women. The lowest proportion of severe ill health is found in the group aged 65 to 69, married, born in Sweden, and having an income in the highest income quintile – 3 per cent among men and 4 per cent among women.

In general women report more problems with health than men, with the exception of hearing problems. Pain is an important factor for older people's experience of health and wellbeing. About 60 per cent of female pensioners and about 40 per cent of male pensioners report pain in at least one body part. The difference is less in the highest age group, mainly because the figure increases more for men. The same picture is valid for mental health problems, although the figures, of course, are lower.

Women of all ages suffer from mental health problems such as anxiety, worry or problems with sleep to a considerably larger extent than men. From the beginning of the 1980s, mild anxiety and worry problems have declined somewhat among women in the 65 to 74 age group and in both sexes in the 75 to 84 age group. The proportion who report severe anxiety or worry problems has remained relatively constant among both sexes during the same period. In 1998/99 about one-third of women and a quarter of men stated that they had sleeping problems.

There is a growing tendency for more and more social categories to be identified as being in need of help from the Swedish welfare system. One such category is older immigrants.

Ronström (2002) argued that public resources are made available to certain categories but only if they accept being identified as a marginalized or problematic group. The acceptance of labelling leads to a strengthening of their marginal position. In 1996, older immigrants made up about 7 per cent of all people 65 and above. It is estimated that this figure will double by the year 2010. Today most of the older immigrants come from neighbouring countries, in particular Finland, but the number who come from further away is increasing rapidly.

Public discussion about older immigrants started in the late 1970s and the first research was published in the early 1980s. According to Ronström, many of the data have been produced by professionals alternating among social administration, social work and research. The research has been initiated and financed by the social authorities. The picture of older immigrants that has been built up over the years is bleak. Health is worse, income is lower, living standards are worse and life expectancy is lower than that of the majority population (Ronström 2002).

Conclusion

The situation for older people in Sweden is generally quite good, measured both objectively and subjectively. Nevertheless, health follows a social gradient and socio-economic differences in health and mortality remain long after retirement.

Overall, self-reported health has improved since the mid-1980s, although the picture is ambiguous. Mobility has improved, the proportion of disabilities has decreased, and the proportion of ADL difficulties has diminished. Despite these advances, no corresponding reduction in the prevalence of long-term illness can be noted and more older people are receiving medical treatment for their long-term illnesses in 2004 than 20 years earlier. Similarly, extended life expectancy since the mid-1980s has not granted additional years free from disease. Most of the increase is made up of years with somewhat impaired health. Finally, up to one in four 70 year olds suffer from serious mental disturbances. Many of these problems in older people are linked to a lifelong psychological vulnerability.

A comparatively high proportion of the older population in Sweden remain in the workforce. Still, the employment rate and retirement age will remain a

SWEDEN: QUALITY OF LIFE IN OLD AGE I

major concern. Efforts to retain these levels, and even to raise them, are coun-
teracted by two forces. On the one hand, ageist norms counter participation in
various activities including work. On the other hand, the interest among older
workers in continuing after the age of 65 is low. There is reason to believe that
economic incentives need to be quite strong to convince people to postpone
retirement. Pensions from work are not the only source of income. Future
generations of older people will possess a high net capital. Consequently, generational transitions through gifts and inheritance could become even more
important than today. All in all, accumulated income is high enough for most
older people to get along quite well, with very few dependant on social assistance – two groups which stand out are older women and newly arrived immigrants who live on the margin.

Housing is a very important aspect of the QoL for older people. They spend
much more time at home than younger individuals. The high standard of
housing for older people in Sweden is an accepted fact. What can be called into
question is the lack of lifts, which will be a major problem for some. The
opportunity to travel is essential for a normal life outdoors. This implies a
need for an effective public transport system; one noteworthy example of such
a system is the service routes. However, being able to come outdoors is not
always enough to facilitate a higher quality of life. An increasing number of
services are being carried out via Web sites. During a transitional period, the
comparatively low access to the Internet among older people can lead to exclusion from central societal functions.

6

The UK: Quality of life in old age I

Alan Walker and Carol Walker[1]

Introduction

Research on QoL in old age has a long tradition in the UK and, in fact, was a key factor in the creation of the discipline of social gerontology. Until recently this research tradition was dominated by health and health-related indicators – such as functional capacity, health status, psychological wellbeing, morale, dependence, coping and adjustment – which have been widely used as proxies for QoL. Within this perspective 'expert' judgements have tended to predominate with little or no reference to the ways in which older people themselves define or understand their own QoL. It is not surprising, therefore, that the dominant scientific and professional approach to researching and assessing QoL in old age has tended to homogenize older people rather than recognizing diversity and differences, based, for example, on age, gender, race and ethnicity, and disability. Recent critiques of this paradigm have resulted in new approaches to the definition and assessment of QoL, which start from the perspective of older people themselves (Bowling 1995; Bond 1999; Grundy and Bowling 1999; Brown *et al.* 2003).

Like the whole of the EU, the UK has an ageing population (Chapter 1). Table 6.1 shows the proportion of the total population made up by different age groups and the predicted expansion in the number of older people that will occur up to 2051. As can be seen, population ageing is expected to continue as the population of young people shrinks and that of older people rises. The trend is a long-term one: at the turn of the twentieth century those aged 65 and over comprised just 4.7 per cent of the population and those aged 80 and over only 0.3 per cent. Presently, there are some 10.8 million people over state pension age (60 for women, 65 for men) and this figure is projected to rise by 11 per cent to 11.9 million by 2011, to 12.3 million by 2021 and to 16 million by 2041 when the median age of the population will be 44.5 years. Without the recent increase in the women's state pension age to 65 this total figure would have been 18 million in 2040.

Hidden within Table 6.1 is one of the most important features of the older population – its gender distribution. At successively older ages the population of women increasingly exceeds that of men. Currently women comprise 49 per cent of those aged 0 to 24, 50 per cent of those aged 25 to 64, 53 per cent of the 65 to 74 age group, 61 per cent of the 75 to 84 age group and 72 per cent of those aged 85 and over. The main reason for disparity in longevity by age is that female life expectancy (at birth) exceeds the male rate by 4.9 years. Largely because of different life expectancies, the majority of men aged 75 and over are married (62 per cent) whereas the majority of women of that age are widowed (64 per cent). These differences are likely to decline along with the disparity in longevity.

Because of the pattern of immigration to the UK, the population of older people in black and ethnic minority groups is currently much smaller than that of the white population – only 6 per cent of black, 7 per cent of Indian, 6 per cent of Chinese and 3 per cent of Pakistani/Bangladeshi groups are over the age of 65 compared with 16 per cent of the white group. Progressive ageing within ethnic minority groups is expected in the future (but depends on fertility levels, mortality rates and net immigration).

Table 6.1 Age groups as a proportion of total UK population (percentages)

Ages	2000	2011	2021	2031	2041	2051
0–14	18.9	16.8	16.2	16.0	15.3	15.3
15–29	19.1	19.6	18.1	16.8	17.2	16.9
30–44	23.0	20.9	19.3	19.5	18.1	18.4
45–59	18.5	20.3	21.3	18.3	19.4	18.6
60–74	13.1	14.9	16.4	18.7	17.1	17.2
75 and over	7.4	7.6	8.6	10.7	13.0	13.6
All ages	100.0	100.0	100.0	100.0	100.0	100.0

Source: Government actuary's mid-2000 based principal projections.

Definition and measurement of quality of life

It is now generally accepted that QoL is a multidimensional concept that does not have clear fixed boundaries (Bond 1999) and that it is best approached in terms of different domains of life (Bowling 1995; Hughes 1990), but there is no agreement about the content of the individual 'domains' of QoL or how to standardize these 'domains' to reflect high or low QoL, or how the relevance of each 'domain' to the individual is to be measured (Brown *et al.* 2003). Thus, according to Bowling (2003):

> Quality of life (QoL) is a multi-level and amorphous concept, and is popular as an endpoint in the evaluation of public policy . . . But the wider research community has accepted no definitive theoretical framework, and no single research framework has been utilized in its investigation. Thus, despite a plethora of research on a wide range of objective and subjective indicators of QoL, there is no widely accepted or supported theory or measurement of QoL.

Some of the problems of defining QoL derive from the need to integrate objective and subjective aspects in a single multidimensional concept. In addition, in interpreting data and designing research instruments, attention must be paid to the significant impact of cultural experience on QoL. Race, gender and class have a powerful determining effect on people's life experience and expectations. So does age: expectations and experiences differ across the generations. Negative approaches to the analysis of old age present a false homogeneity among older people as a social group. The idea of old age as a leveller has become an obstruction to understanding economic and social conditions as causes of poor QoL in old age (Walker 1980, 1993). More recent developments in the theorizing of QoL recognize this diversity among older people and the multifaceted nature of ageing (Hughes 1990; Bowling 1995; Grundy and Bowling 1999).

A common characteristic of different disciplinary approaches to QoL is that concepts have been based on 'expert' opinions rather than those of lay people (Rogerson *et al.* 1989) and it is only very recently that the focus has been shifted from the former to the latter. Thus path-breaking research undertaken for the GO programme (Bowling *et al.* 2002) set out to explore older people's own definitions of, and priorities for, a good QoL. The majority of people rated their QoL as good in varying degrees, with almost three-quarters of those in the 65 to 69 group rating their lives overall as 'So good it could not be better' or 'Very good'. Half those in the older age groups gave similarly positive responses.

The main elements that older people identified as being important to their QoL were:

- people's standards of social comparison and expectations in life;

- a sense of optimism and belief that 'all will be well in the end' rather than a tendency to think the worst;

- having good health and physical functioning;

- engaging in a large number of social activities and feeling supported;

- living in a neighbourhood with good community facilities and services, including transport;

- feeling safe in one's neighbourhood.

Having a sense of control over one's life was reported as a mediating variable. The researchers concluded that these factors contributed far more to perceived QoL than indicators of material circumstances, such as actual level of income, education, home ownership, or social class. Using three different research methods, the conclusions show a high level of consensus among older people about what makes a good QoL. The study also confirmed how the various factors interact so that deterioration in one area, such as health, could have a domino effect on other factors such as social interaction and independence.

Age Concern England has suggested that government should adopt a strategic approach to meeting older people's needs based on the evidence produced by the various research projects undertaken for the GO Programme and should take account of the interdependence of those determinants (Bowling 2003a). Given that QoL is 'inherently a dynamic, multi-level and complex concept, reflecting objective, subjective, macro-societal, and micro-individual, positive and negative influences which interact together' (Lawton 1991, cited in Bowling 2003: 46) debates on its definition and measurement are set to continue. However, there is a need to combine the quantitative measures which have predominated in much health-oriented research with more qualitative work that puts older people at the centre of determining what makes up and impacts upon a good QoL.

Environments of ageing

The majority of older people live in their own homes and the proportion of both men and women continues to rise up to the age of 79 but then falls slightly for men and significantly for women over the age of 80, as more move into alternative supported living or residential care settings (see Table 6.2).

House ownership is often used as an indicator of wealth. However, the data on housing tenures of older people do not reveal their standard of living: the house-owning ageing population includes a large proportion of households that are equity rich and income poor. The responsibility for maintaining a property grows while incomes remain fixed. Fifteen per cent of those older people who live independently in their own homes live in housing that is in poor condition, either needing modernization or in a state of serious disrepair. These people are more likely to be over 70 years of age (DoE 2001). Female-headed households experience some of the worst housing conditions across the lifecourse and it is likely that they will continue to figure disproportionately as they and their properties age (Leather 1998).

Table 6.2 Housing tenure, by age and sex

	50–4	55–9	60–4	65–9	70–4	75–9	80+	Total
Men								
Owned outright	27.5	37.8	55.9	70.8	72.9	73.1	66.9	53.2
Buying with mortgage/ Shared ownership	59.1	46.6	27.3	10.1	6.8	5.4	4.0	28.7
Renting	13.4	15.6	16.8	19.1	20.3	21.5	29.0	18.1
Women								
Owned outright	32.5	47.5	65.1	73.6	67.8	65.2	59.1	56.7
Buying with mortgage/ Shared ownership	50.7	39.1	20.7	9.6	6.6	5.6	4.6	22.3
Renting	16.8	13.4	14.2	16.8	25.6	29.1	36.3	21.0

Source: Marmot *et al.* (2003, Table 8A.1).

Thus home ownership offers both advantages and disadvantages to older people and can be experienced both as a benefit and as a burden (Askham *et al.* 1999):

♦ independence: having control over their future and their homes, but also having to deal with repairs and maintenance;

♦ finance: the home is a capital asset, offers security for the future and is cheaper than renting, but the property might have to be sold to pay for institutional care later and there is little help available with housing or repair costs;

♦ identity: many see themselves as people with responsibility and moral worth, hard working and secure achievers, but also as tied down, responsible for growing maintenance and repairs, with many worries and responsibilities not shared by tenants.

'Architectural disability' is a term used to describe the ways the physical design and construction of buildings can form barriers for people, making the built environment uncomfortable and unsafe for people to use. Architectural disability is mainly caused by small spaces and difficult changes of level (Peace and Holland 2001a). Design flaws in the built environment can cause inequality by denying access to buildings, and lowering people's self-esteem by discrimination, which happens to people from all walks of life, mothers with young children in pushchairs, older people, tall, short or disabled people. Most houses in which older people live present difficulties as they grow older. Many are unsuitable for adaptation. Houses might be too big, expensive to run, in a wrong location or inconvenient, especially if the owner is no longer able to drive. Thus some older people feel constrained by their housing environment and see it as disabling. Those with sufficient means can enjoy specially designed environments but others will stay trapped in architecturally disabling housing if they do not have access to appropriate housing conditions which meet their changing needs and capacities (Hanson 2001). Although there is a system for assisting older people to obtain the necessary aids and adaptations in their own homes (whether owned or rented), local authority budgets for this are extremely limited and there are often delays in having the work done (Table 6.3). Because of tight financial limits major works are particularly difficult to obtain and there are variations between areas.

One of the problems older people have to face when living independently is the poor design of most of the housing stock in the UK, which is often built on several levels, making negotiating stairs a necessity. Each year there are over a million accidents resulting from falls, which are non-fatal, but a quarter of them are serious and, of these, almost half involve people over 65 years old. In the three year period 1995–97 there were nearly 2250 deaths of people over 75 years old due to falls at home; two-thirds were women (Department of Trade and Industry 1999). The types of fatal falls involving people over 65 were divided as follows: 62 per cent fell on the stairs or from a stepladder, 15 per cent fell between two levels (from a chair or bed), 13 per cent on the same level, 6 per cent from a ladder and 4 per cent from a building.

133

Table 6.3 Adaptations to accommodation, by age and sex

	60–64	65–9	70–4	75–9	80+	Total 50+
Men						
Widened halls/doorways	14.1	9.8	12.8	5.1	7.0	10.9
Handrails	61.4	59.3	64.6	62.1	62.6	59.3
Bathroom modifications	37.4	45.9	44.6	54.0	53.9	45.4
Chairlift/stair glide	6.3	7.1	4.7	7.1	9.9	6.8
Women						
Widened halls/doorways	12.7	11.8	9.2	9.8	5.7	10.0
Handrails	51.3	60.5	61.0	60.6	60.5	58.3
Bathroom modifications	43.0	50.9	48.2	52.4	52.2	48.7
Chairlift/stair glide	4.9	5.5	7.9	11.0	11.8	8.6

Source: Marmot *et al.* (2003, Table 8A.7).

Special housing and institutional care

About 5 per cent of older people live in residential care homes (DoE 2001). In England there are about 476,000 units of sheltered accommodation and 23,000 very sheltered housing units. The total number of people over state pension age living in communal residential and nursing care homes in 2000 was 350,000 (TSO 2002). Unsurprisingly the chances of living in a care home or nursing home increase as people get older. In 1998, 0.5 per cent of under 65 year olds lived in such accommodation compared to 1 per cent for people aged 65 to 74, 5 per cent for people aged 75 to 84 years and 21.7 per cent for those over 85 years old (Laing and Buisson 1999).

Often the decision about a change in accommodation is made under stress when the current living arrangements break down, usually due to illness or increased frailty. The decision may be taken on frail older people's behalf. A key element that influences people's feelings of wellbeing is the extent to which they feel in control of their decisions and manage their activities of daily living. Residential care represents a loss of independence and autonomy. Moving into a residential or nursing home also has profound implications for the financial situation of older people and often their families, as charges increasingly exceed the limits that are met by the government and local authorities. Many older people in the UK are reluctant to move into residential care or nursing homes because it means losing their own home and all the associations and memories associated with it. Research by Peace and her colleagues (2003) found that many objects in people's homes were significant for self-identity. Limited personal possessions can, of course, accompany the person into residential care but Peace *et al.* (2003) found that equally important were such things as long-tended gardens with favourite plants, views from certain windows, familiar walks, none of which are transportable. Many people living in residential care settings always feel as if they are 'living in someone else's home' (Clough 1996).

At present residential care is seen as having several groups of stakeholders: residents, advocates and relatives; staff delivering care; investors, regulators, contractors and society as potential users. The principle of empowerment of both residents and staff in residential care has been accepted increasingly since the end of the 1980s. However, putting it into practice and actually influencing the nature of care still has a long way to go (Peace *et al.* 1997). Residential care has changed significantly since the mid-1980s as government policy has moved local authorities from being providers to purchasers of such care for older people. The majority of residential accommodation is now provided by the private and voluntary sectors. More sophisticated inspections and co-ordination with the Social Services Inspectorate have been developed (Peace *et al.* 1997) but the ideal of a small 'homely' home rarely exists and the large 'warehouse' is increasingly common.

Tune and Bowie (2000) present a more optimistic picture. Out of 46 residential and nursing homes they examined, 94 per cent were said to be 'resident-orientated' rather than 'institution-orientated'. In the former category more flexible patterns of care had been implemented offering more personal choice and more respect for individuals. This represents a notable improvement over previous findings. According to this study the physical condition of local authority homes was poorer than privately run homes and some improvements could be made without major cost implications.

Despite the negative views held of residential care by those outside the system, residents interviewed in a small residential home reported positive aspects to their environment. They felt secure and liked the fact that they did not have to engage with other people more than they wanted to. Some residents developed real friendships with others but mostly the atmosphere among residents could best be described as tolerance and polite interest (Peace and Holland 2001b). Proprietors described their relationships in some cases with great affection and generally as good.

Residential and nursing homes have dominated the delivery of long-term care for older people in the UK. Retirement communities could challenge this domination if they could deliver the same level of care at a similar or reduced cost. The best argument for retirement communities lies in their claim to increase the QoL for their residents. Kingston *et al.* (2001) looked at two groups of older people, one living in a retirement community in the West Midlands and the other attending local day centres run by charities. The mean age of the retirement community group was 80.1 and community sample group 76.4. The retirement community residents scored significantly higher in terms of both mental and general health. During the year of this study the older people in the retirement community maintained their health status and it became clear that their self-reported health status had been very stable, whereas the local community sample had a more variable self-reported health status. The main reasons given for moving into a retirement community were security and a way of ensuring they did not become a burden on their family. The researchers reported that those living in the retirement community experienced camaraderie and support from other tenants, and a sense of optimism stemming from the neighbourliness and security of their surroundings, which contributed to their wellbeing.

About 5 per cent of older people live in sheltered or very sheltered accommodation. Sheltered housing has been developed as a resource for older people to meet their changing housing needs – it is usually fully accessible – and their low levels of support needs. Sheltered housing allows people to live fully independently but within a communal setting. It has been found to offer a sense of security, especially if there is resident warden and contact with other people (Nocon and Peace 1999). In these communal environments older people find it easy to meet people, form new networks and friendship groups and receive support within an age-segregated environment (Percival 2001). But sheltered housing can also weaken positive feelings and exacerbate negative attitudes, experiences and behaviours, causing intolerance and frustration. When a sheltered housing environment was socially vibrant and balanced in terms of the levels of disability of its tenants, satisfaction was high, but living along with frail older people might emphasize the negative side of ageing to younger socially oriented tenants (Oldman 2000). Friction can occur between different groups of tenants.

National Health Service geriatric beds have reduced in number since the early 1970s from about 400,000 to 190,000 in 2000 and current government policy is to end 'bed blocking' by getting older people who need only nursing care out of hospital into the community. Penalties are now imposed on Social Services Departments who do not provide a community place within a specified period. Concomitantly there has also been a dramatic growth in the independent (mostly private) nursing home industry, which has grown from 28,000 beds in 1983 to 196,000 in 1999 (in England). Over half of all health-care beds are now in nursing homes in England, which means that large parts of the UK healthcare sector have been privatized. In the Care Standards Act 2000, regulatory jurisdiction was given to the new National Care Standards Commission over care services including care homes. This Act has been criti-cized for being based on a 'command and control' principle and to overcome this it is suggested that public interest groups should be involved to increase the accountability of the industry and the regulator (Kerrison and Pollock 2001). In the case of nursing homes, such public interest groups could include residents or their relatives or representatives from voluntary organizations, who could be consulted about the standards used in regulating the nursing homes. 'Fit for Future', which was compiled by a range of voluntary agencies (Department of Health 1999), put forward recommendations for national standards for care homes for older people, but these are currently only for guidance and are not legally enforceable. Staffing levels in care homes are the most important factor in ensuring good quality of care, but as at 2004 the government has not imposed staffing ratios for care homes.

The movement of older people from NHS beds, which are free, to nursing homes, which are means tested, has created a situation where one in every three residents of care homes pay the whole of their fees. It has been argued that residents should, therefore, be seen as consumers instead of residents and, in this way, be covered by consumer legislation. Moreover, introducing a regulator to this sector will enforce the human and consumer rights of people who might be too frail to protect themselves. When the Office of Fair Trading looked into contracts between residents and care homes they found that many of these contravened regulations on unfair terms and only one in five residents even knew they had a contract with the care home (Kerrison and Pollock 2001). Greater user involvement might encourage the enforcement of regulations.

Crime and the fear of crime

Statistically, older people are less likely to become victims of crime than are younger people (Carvel 2001). Nonetheless, crime is frequently raised by older people as being a major concern for them and they are often reported in the UK media as being very fearful of crime. From the British Crime Survey it is evident that women on the whole worry more about crime than men (Table 6.4). Of the people who were very worried about crime, older women

Table 6.4 Fear of crime:[1] by gender and age 2000

England and Wales	Males				Females			
	16–29	30–59	60 and over	All aged 16 and over	16–29	30–59	60 and over	All aged 16 and over
Theft of car[2]	22	18	19	19	27	21	21	22
Theft from car[2]	19	16	15	16	18	15	15	16
Burglary	17	16	15	16	23	21	22	22
Mugging	12	10	12	11	24	21	25	23
Physical attack	11	8	8	9	33	26	23	27
Rape	12	7	4	7	37	29	24	29

1 Percentage of people who were 'very worried' about each type of crime.
2 Percentage of car owners.
Source: British Crime Survey, Home Office (2000).

are most likely to worry about muggings; younger women worry more about physical attacks, burglaries and car theft than either older women or men.

A number of explanations have been offered for older people's fear of crime being greater than their actual experience of crime. These include the dispro-portionate impact on health given the time it may take to recover from a phys-ical attack and the extra vulnerability older people feel as they are unable to run away from younger, fitter attackers. It has been argued that older people's fear of crime should be seen in the context of social isolation and the process of deskilling in relation to their environment (Jones 1987). Older people living in deprived areas are likely to be more fearful of crime. An opinion poll, pub-lished by Help the Aged, found that the most vulnerable group of older people were living on incomes of less than £6,500 per year. In their study of older people in deprived neighbourhoods, Scharf and colleagues (2003) found that 40 per cent of respondents had been the victim of one or more types of crime in the preceding two years. Only 7 per cent said they would feel safe leaving their home after dark compared to 44 per cent who said they would feel very unsafe. This sense of insecurity in a neighbourhood obviously restricts older people's ability to participate in social activities. Poorer older people who do not have access to a car are even more likely to be restricted in participating in evening activities. Concern about personal safety is a major barrier to many older people using public transport, especially in the evening or at night. Gilhooly's (2003) GO research found this fear extended not only to riding on buses or trains but also to safety while waiting and while walking to and from the stops and stations. Two-thirds of the older people taking part in this study said that concerns about personal safety (in the evening or at night) was a barrier to using public transport.

Technology

Technology is intergenerational because it has the ability to improve the QoL for all people (Bernard and Phillips 2000). It has the potential to assist people who have limited mobility, for example, by easing communication difficulties, overcoming barriers created by poor house design, shopping, voting, obtaining information, claiming benefits and so on. Providing enabling communications systems can give people from different ages, gender and ethnic minority groups the opportunity to continue to participate as citizens within their local communities. Technology can play a part in overcoming longstanding barriers in conventional policy areas such as housing, education, social services, and health to create a 'seamless' service (Griffiths 1988).

New technologies, such as robotics, telecommunications, telematics and information processing will have a significant future impact on community care for older people. The scope is increasing for new technology to assist older people in every day living tasks, such as mobility, preparing meals and ensuring personal hygiene (Sixsmith 1994). Technological communication links could enable more older people to remain at home by facilitating remote monitoring by service providers. This would allow more people to enjoy independent living in circumstances where they currently might have to move into care homes or hospitals. Monitoring systems using video links and optical fibres are less intrusive and reduce information processing on the service provider (Sixsmith 1994). New technologies could make it possible for service providers to deliver more flexible and good quality community and healthcare and respond to individual preferences and lifestyle requirements that would reduce isolation and enhance feelings of autonomy, security and safety. All these factors would delay dependency and give economic viability to the development of these technologies. For example, traditional alarm systems used in many older people's homes and sheltered housing accommodation, which rely on the older person being able to raise the alarm, can be replaced by new infrared sensors that detect movement and which automatically raise the alarm if movement is not detected over a set period.

Technology can be used to reduce the social exclusion of older people and mobility-impaired groups by helping them to find their way in the built environment (Hine *et al.* 2000). The use of new technology, specifically personal computers and access to the Internet, is now widespread in the UK and a minority of older people take advantage of this. It is estimated that in the UK there are over 4.6 million computer users over 50 who spend about 9 hours a week at their computers and 2.2 million older people regularly surf the Internet. A special chat room created by Age Concern (www.bbb.org.uk) has been running since 1999 and is used by about 4000 older people.

However, although the 2002 ELSA (English Longitudinal Study of Ageing) sweep found that overall 48.4 of men and 38.6 of women over 50 own a computer, this figure falls dramatically as people age (Marmot *et al.* 2003). Thus, among men this figure falls to 29.1 per cent in the 70 to 74 age group, 19.7 per cent for those 75 to 79, 12.2 per cent 80+. Among women, the proportions for the same age groups are 21.5 per cent, 14.9 per cent and 6.0 per cent respectively. Of course older people who do not have access to the Internet from home can access it from local libraries, Age Resource Centres and elsewhere but lack of ownership in this case is likely to be due to unfamiliarity and fear of new technology, not just ability to pay. Thus, while making information available online is an important resource, it cannot yet replace traditional forms of communication for older people. This is particularly the case for government departments, including social security, which are increasingly encouraging people to download information and application forms from the Internet.

Transport

Access to transport, public or private, is crucial for older people's participation in everyday activities outside the home. For many it becomes a more significant issue when they cannot walk very far or carry heavy shopping bags. For some, physical impairment may mean that they have to give up a private car and use public transport. A major survey of people aged 60 and over revealed that where older people have access to a car, it is their first choice of transport. For other people, buses are most frequently used. Many people, especially those with disabilities, use taxis, which suggests that community and public transport do not meet their needs. One-third of participants reported that they were unable to undertake one or more activities as often as they wanted because of transport problems. For half of these respondents this meant they were unable to make social visits to see family and friends. Older people with sensory impairments and those over 80 are constrained in their ability to travel because of limited mobility. Transport needs to be both readily available and accessible to meet their needs.

One in eight of the people interviewed said they would like to see their families more often, of whom 58 per cent said they did not do so because of public transport-related difficulties such as cost, difficulties boarding and leaving the vehicle, the bus stop being too far away, transport being too unreliable, the journey being too uncomfortable or public transport being confusing to use. A small number wanted to attend a local day centre but were unable to because of transport difficulties. Eight per cent of respondents wanted to undertake more leisure and sporting activities but 57 per cent of these said they could not because of lack of transport. Carrying heavy shopping is a major problem for older people without a car.

Gilhooly et al.'s GO research (2003) set out to test whether the widely held assertion that accessible public transport and the independence that is associated with car driving are indeed linked to QoL. The study concluded that both were found to be independent predictors of QoL and demonstrated that good access to transport itself is associated with higher perceived QoL. This was quite separate from the impact of income and wealth as measured by car ownership.

Where older people still own and can drive a car, then they tend to use it as their main form of transport. Gilhooly et al.'s (2003) study identified four types of 'car access' in relation to QoL: household car ownership, car driving, ease of access as a driver, and ease of access to a car as a passenger. All types of car access were found to be associated with higher perceived QoL. All respondents who owned a car reported that it enhanced their QoL because it enabled them to lead fuller lives and allowed them to reach all desired locations. Driving was more closely associated with QoL by men than women. The researchers attribute this to the status that men derive from car ownership. Thus they found that, while there was no difference in QoL between female drivers and non-drivers, there was a difference for men. As higher proportions of drivers age, the prospect of having to give up driving is becoming a reality for more and more older people. Gilhooly et al. (2003: 2) found that:

> Persuading drivers to discuss giving up driving, and the circumstances under which they might do so, proved to be remarkably difficult. Having to give up driving was so clearly associated with anticipated problems of getting about, as well as with negative perceptions of old age, that most people said they could not bring themselves to actively plan for such an eventuality.

However, contrary to the fears of current drivers, this study also found that older people who had already given up driving were less negative. While they did report a loss of freedom as the main disadvantage, they also reported fewer problems in using public transport or continuing with activities than were anticipated by current drivers.

Public transport is of particular significance for older people; the majority are women who, especially among older generations, are less likely to be able to drive and many drivers will have to give up their cars because of physical impairment or on financial grounds. While Gilhooly and her colleagues (2003) found that greater satisfaction with public transport was associated with QoL, the correlations were low, indicating that only a small proportion of the variance in reported QoL could be attributed to satisfaction with public transport. Nevertheless, respondents reported that they thought improvements in public transport would improve their QoL. In a government study on the transport needs of older people (DETLGR 2001), older people made several suggestions for improving public transport including improvements in reliability, improved timetabling, introducing penalties for service operators for failures in service, and the reintroduction of bus conductors, which would control bad behaviour by passengers and therefore improve security.

A number of studies have sought to explore the barriers to the use of public transport. The 2002 ELSA research highlighted six possible explanations: too expensive (55.7 per cent of all men over 50, 53.2 per cent of all women over 50), too unreliable (57.6 per cent for men, 54.5 per cent for women), too infrequent (57.1 per cent and 55.4 per cent respectively), health prevents them (54.7 per cent and 53.8 per cent), do not need to use it (54.7 per cent and 53.8 per cent), there is none available (84.8 per cent and 83.1 per cent). The proportion reporting the above factors as a barrier to public transport use increased consistently with age. The proportion of people reporting the unavailability of public transport is of particular concern and can only be resolved by a coherent national transport policy that takes account of the social needs of people rather than just the economic cost of providing transport services. Surprisingly, the ELSA study does not report security as a separate category although the majority of respondents (59.6 per cent for men and 56.4 per cent for women overall, rising to 71.7 per cent and 79.4 among the over 80 age group) gave 'other reasons' for not using public transport. As previously noted, studies of crime frequently report that security is a major issue in deterring older people from using public transport at night. This was also the reason most frequently given by respondents in Gilhooly et al.'s (2003) research (65 per cent).

Transport is a particular issue for older people living in rural areas, where petrol tends to be more expensive and public transport limited (Farrington 1999). Bus services are very restricted in most rural areas, with just one or two services a day and distances to essential services, for example in the nearest town, can be considerable (Wenger 2001). People living in rural areas may not benefit from the free bus passes available to most older people living in cities (Wenger 2001). Few rural communities are served by a train service; few have a railway station (Wenger 1984). Inability or reluctance to use public transport means that people become more socially isolated; they are unable to visit family and friends as often as they would like, participation in clubs and day centres is limited, and it may be difficult to see the doctor or go to the nearest hospital.

A brief glimpse into the attitudes of public transport providers in Gilhooley et al.'s (2003) study is not encouraging. Only one-third of older people thought that bus operators considered the needs of older people; two-thirds thought that train operators did. Confidential interviews with operators revealed that disability, not ageing, was the prime concern and disability was, as is often the case, interpreted in terms of wheelchair accessibility. Few mentioned the needs of those with sensory impairments, which particularly affect older people. The researchers refer to off-the-record remarks that indicated that transport operators regarded older people as a 'nuisance', which they say might be attributed to the perception that free or concessionary fares reduce profit margins. Conversely, and for obvious commercial reasons, car manufacturers were found to be thinking seriously about the ageing of the population and how to make car driving easier and safer for older people.

Physical and mental health

General Household Survey (GHS) data reveal that 22 per cent of men and 21 per cent of women between the ages of 65 and 74 reported poor general health in 2000–1. This rose to 29 per cent and 26 per cent respectively in the 75 and over age group (TSO 2002). A longstanding illness was reported by 61 per cent of men and 54 per cent of men in the lower age group and 63 per cent and 64 per cent respectively among the older age group (TSO 2002).

Failing health or disability is a major reason for older people moving into some form of residential care. In 2000, 82 per cent of older people living in residential care reported a longstanding illness or disability compared to 69 per cent of those living in their own home (Health Survey for England

2000). Locomotor disability was the most frequently reported disability reported by those in care homes (65 per cent), whereas only 10 per cent of older people living in their own households reported this kind of impairment. Fifty-four per cent of people in care homes reported serious restrictions regarding their own personal care compared to only 3 per cent among those living in households. Older women are much more likely to experience restrictions to their mobility, their ability to perform household tasks and self-care than older men. In some cases twice as many women than men were unable to walk down the road unaided or to go up or down stairs. Nearly half of women over 85 were unable to walk down the road unaided, whereas less than one-fifth of men over 85 were unable to do so (Arber and Cooper 1999). Older women experience more disadvantage than older men because of more severe disability and often more isolated living arrangements. Older men with a disability, unlike older women, are more likely to have a spouse to provide care for them and are therefore less likely to have to rely on friends and neighbours, domiciliary services or to enter residential care. Sixty per cent of older women with moderate or severe disability live alone, relying on family, friends or neighbours to give assistance when needed to enable them to remain living at home. If these forms of assistance were not available they would need to have home care services or move to a care home. Income is an issue on entry to residential care: older people with only the state pension to rely on are more likely to enter residential care than people with middle incomes. Older women are more likely to report poor health because they are more likely to be socially and financially disadvantaged than old men (Arber and Cooper 1999).

Older people are two to three times more likely to be depressed than to have dementia. Depression is not part of normal ageing or age-related but it is more common among older people who are physically ill (Anderson 2001) and yet ELSA findings (Marmot *et al.* 2003, table 6A.14) show that there is a decrease in diagnosed mental illness with age (which is attributed to the possibility of happy people living longer). Older people with Parkinson's disease, stroke, neurological disorders or dementia have higher rates of depression. Depression without treatment easily becomes a chronic disorder producing high levels of mortality and morbidity. In later life depression is a largely untreated and undetected condition (Anderson 2001) and yet older depressed people will visit their GP two to three times more often than older people with no depression.

Many studies agree that a factor that can increase the chances of experiencing depression is deteriorating physical health and functional capacity in later years and that support from family members and confidants can provide some protection against it. People with low coping resources, such as economic difficulties, are also more likely to report depression (Silveira and Alleback 2001). The limited research that has been done with older people in migrant groups reveals that they have fewer resources to cope with problems, which may lead to mental health problems. Silveira and Alleback (2001), for example, looked at the Somali elders in Tower Hamlets in London, interviewing 28 Somali men aged over 60. The main causes of depression among this group of older people included decreased mobility and pain, life-threatening illnesses and inadequate access to services (which the authors found to be greater for this group than the general population), breakdown in social support, feelings of deprivation, loss of work roles, ageism as well as loss of family members in the civil war in their home country and the long distance from their family, economic losses there (including property), the need to support relatives who were left behind, and immigration and citizenship issues (Silveira and Allebeck 2001).

Employment and retirement

In common with most other EU countries there is a well-entrenched trend towards early exit from the UK labour market, particularly among men. Since the 1950s there has been a dramatic fall in the proportion of economically active men aged 55 and over in the UK, a process that continued, then levelled out during the 1990s and, very recently, has shown an upward trend (Table 6.5). The picture for women is less clear but, once the cohort effect of the post-war rise in female economic activity is disentangled from the cross-sectional picture shown in Table 6.5, a similar but less sharp trend can be observed among older women (Guillemard 1993).

The main factors explaining the growth of early exit from the UK labour market are demand related, particularly the recessions of the mid-1970s and early 1980s (Walker 1985; Trinder 1990). There are three main reasons for the decline in economic activity among older people. First, older workers are over-represented in declining industries, such as primary industries and manufacturing, and under-represented in growing ones. Second, older workers are both more likely to be made redundant than younger ones and subsequently less likely to find alternative employment. Third, for an organization wanting to shed staff quickly, it is relatively easy to negotiate early retirement for those close to pension age (Taylor and Walker 1996). Thus, rather than being a trend based on personal preferences for early retirement on the part of older workers

145

Table 6.5 Labour force participation of older men and women in Britain 1951–2000

	1951	1961	1971	1975	1981	1985	1991	1995	1998	2000
Age group:										
Men										
55–9	95.0	97.1	95.3	93.0	89.4	82.0	80.6	73.7	74.5	74.8
60–4	87.7	91.0	86.6	82.3	69.3	54.4	54.1	50.1	49.5	50.3
65+	31.1	25.0	23.5	19.2	10.3	8.2	8.6	8.2	7.6	7.9
Women										
55–9	29.1	39.2	50.9	52.4	53.4	52.1	54.3	55.7	54.6	57.6
60–4	14.1	19.7	28.8	28.6	23.3	18.9	23.9	25.0	23.7	25.9
65+	4.6	6.3	4.9	3.7	3.0	3.3	3.1	3.2	3.4	3.4

Sources: 1951–71 Census of Population for England and Wales and for Scotland; 1975–2000 Department of Employment, Gazette (various); UK Labour Force Survey.

(though of course some do exercise such a preference) the research evidence shows that the decline in employment was the decisive factor. It has been argued, therefore, that early retirement in the UK is best understood as a form of unemployment (Casey and Laczko 1989).

Despite tightening labour markets in the late 1990s and skills shortages within certain sectors – notably distribution and consumer services, transport and public administration, and in business services (DfEE 1991) – labour force participation among the over-50s continued to decline. Cohort analysis of Labour Force Survey data between 1979 and 1997 indicates that each successive generation of older men has lower employment rates than the preceding one. There is a strong possibility that the next generation of men will stop work even earlier than the current generation and women will exit from the labour force earlier than they would have done had men's effective retirement age not fallen (Campbell 1999). As well as experiencing a disproportionate decline in employment, older men also receive relatively low wages.

Economic activity rates among the over-50s are markedly lower than for those aged under 50. Although older workers are less likely to be unemployed than those aged under 40, once they become unemployed they are more likely to experience longer periods out of work than other age groups; and, as rates of economic activity decline after the age of 50, so too do gross weekly earnings, after peaking during the 40s (Tillsley 1995). Compared with the earnings of men in their mid-40s, average wages for older men have not increased as much in real terms. However, this can only be partially explained by differences in levels of qualifications between these two groups.

Compared with younger workers, older workers in employment are more likely to work on a self-employed basis and to work in part-time jobs. Those working past state pension age are most likely to be in temporary jobs (Tillsley 1995; McKay and Middleton 1998). There is a concentration of older workers, particularly men and women in their early 50s, in manufacturing and other services. With regard to occupations, men aged 45 to 59 are concentrated in management, clerical and craft occupations, whereas among those aged 60 and over there is a move towards working in personal and security occupations and in 'other occupations'. Among women aged 45 to 54, a significant proportion (three in ten) are engaged in clerical and secretarial work, and personal and protective occupations, while among those aged 55 to 64 there is a noticeable growth in working in personal and protective work and 'other occupations' such as cleaning.

Age discrimination

Research on older workers has found evidence of discrimination in all areas of employment. For example, a survey carried out among managers found that 36 per cent reported that there was an age barrier for internal promotions in their organization, while 45 per cent had received no professional development in the last five years (Lewis and McLaverty 1991). Similarly, Ginn and Arber (1996) found that 64 per cent of women and 66 per cent of men aged 40 or over cited their age as the major barrier to obtaining a better job. In addition, a survey conducted of older men's and women's experiences in the labour market (Taylor and Walker 1991, 1996) found that some non-working older workers felt that they had already effectively retired despite being aged in their 50s or early 60s and had become resigned to the fact that they would not work again after discouragement from employers and representatives of official agencies. Age restrictions in job advertisements were frequently cited as barriers to employment. The age of the person doing the interview was also reported as a factor in being turned down for jobs. A greater number of potential working years, 'paper' qualifications and greater adaptability were cited as some reasons why employers would be more likely to employ younger people, although the older workers felt they were more reliable. Another strong feeling was that employers would not wish to train older workers. Several respondents felt that the only jobs open to them were part-time and/or extremely low paid.

A case study of the BBC – the public service broadcaster – illustrates the exclusion of people over 50. In 1978, 900 BBC staff were over 60, which was 3.4 per cent of the workforce and by 1993 only 0.35 per cent of the staff were over 60. While people of 50 years old and over were occupying more than one-fifth of all staff positions in the BBC in 1978, by 1993 this figure had fallen to one-tenth, which makes the BBC a youth-dominated enterprise (Platman and Tinker 1998). Younger people occupied jobs in finance, policy and personnel as well as departments involved in programme output to such an extent that in the core sector no one reached the retirement age of 60 in 1993. The core staff composition is most important in creative output, customer relations and responsiveness. As an organization the BBC has a unique role in customer service; it has taken steps to reflect its audience in terms of race, gender and disability but people over the age of 50 have become excluded from the organization.

Given the existence of age discrimination in the UK labour market, it is not surprising that older non-employed workers have a negative perception of their own labour market position in terms of the probability of them regaining employment (Laczko 1987a) and, as a result, may prefer to define themselves as disabled or early retired (Rosenblum 1975; Walker 1985; Piachaud 1986; Bytheway 1987; Laczko 1987b). Research indicates that older workers have a realistic perception of their prospects for re-employment. For example, Westergaard *et al.* (1989: 64) found that, even within the same socio-economic group, older workers were more likely than younger ones to be unemployed 6 months and 3 years after redundancy. Similarly, Love and Torrence (1989) found that, following plant closures, as well as taking longer to find employment older workers earned less on re-employment than younger workers.

Becoming retired

Increasingly proportions of men and women are retiring before they reach the state retirement age (65 for men and 60 for women). Table 6.6 shows economic activity varies substantially by gender and by age. The significantly higher proportion of women than men who are in part-time work up until retirement

Table 6.6 Primary activity status, by age and gender

	50–4	55–9	60–4	65–9	70–4	75–9	80+
Economically active men	83.3	72.9	48.3	16.5	10.8	5.1	1.1
Economically active women	75.5	61.3	30.3	13.1	4.1	1.6	0.4

Source: Marmot *et al.* (2003), Table 4.1.

age is not shown in the table. However, thereafter there are considerably higher fractions of part-time work for both men and women.

The very high levels of early retirement pose important questions for policy. The 2002 ELSA study (Marmot *et al.* 2003) offers the first national evidence on the push and pull factors that influence decisions on early retirement. The 2002 wave found that both self-reported employment status and labour-market participation rates were lower for individuals in poorer health. Men under the age of 65, the official retirement age, who said that they were in excellent, very good or good health were between 35 and 40 percentage points more likely to be economically active than those in fair or poor health. For women under the age of 60, their official retirement age, the gap was between 30 and 40 percentage points. The ELSA study also found that 'early retirement' is also closely correlated with wealth, with the proportion retired among the highest wealth quintiles being significantly higher than among the lower wealth groups. Future income is also a pull factor when older people are considering early retirement. The 2002 ELSA study also showed the importance of pensions in retirement decisions. One-third of those with private pensions who retired before the normal retirement age in their pension plan reported that they were offered reasonable financial terms to do so and that this was relevant to their retirement decision. Table 6.7 shows the different reasons people gave for retiring before the state retirement age. Over one-quarter of men and women did so because of ill health and just under one-quarter of men and one in eight women did so because they were made redundant, had no choice, or could not find another job.

A small number of studies have examined the factors influencing early retirement decisions but there is a lack of information on the major differences that may exist between people in different occupations or socio-economic groups, as well as differences based on gender or ethnicity. Some insight into the general area of decision making on early retirement is provided by one study of largely male employees, working at different levels within a multi-national company, across several UK plants (Maule *et al.* 1996). More than two-thirds of respondents (70 per cent) identified pension arrangements and lump sum payments as being the most important factors in the decision to take early retirement, while around one in four (24 per cent) were concerned about ill health and future health. Although the survey findings are consistent with those from previous studies (Myers 1983; McGoldrick and Cooper 1988) in identifying finance as being of primary importance in the early retirement decision, Maule *et al.* (1986) highlight the significance of other factors in the

Table 6.7 Reasons for retirement prior to reaching state pension age

Percentage reporting reason for retirement	All individuals	
	Retired before SPA	Retired at or after SPA
Men		
Reached retirement age	7.7	75.1
Own ill health	27.1	6.6
Made redundant/dismissed/had no choice/ could not find another job	23.6	6.7
Offered reasonable financial terms to retire early or take voluntary redundancy	23.2	1.9
Fed up with job and wanted a change	8.0	3.6
To enjoy life while still young and fit enough	17.3	8.9
To spend more time with partner/family	6.6	5.3
Ill health of a relative/friend	5.2	1.7
To retire at the same time as husband/wife/ partner	1.7	1.4
Other	9.9	8.9
Women		
Reached retirement age	2.1	58.3
Own ill health	26.2	10.0
Made redundant/dismissed/had no choice/ could not find another job	14.1	7.8
Offered reasonable financial terms to retire early or take voluntary redundancy	7.7	0.8
Fed up with job and wanted a change	8.1	5.6
To enjoy life while still young and fit enough	13.8	11.2
To spend more time with partner/family	19.1	9.5
Ill health of a relative/friend	11.3	4.4
To retire at the same time as husband/wife/ partner	7.9	5.7
Other	16.6	10.6
Sample size:		
Men	1762	923
Women	1333	1610

Note: respondents were asked to report all relevant reasons for retirement.
Source: Marmot *et al.* (2003, Table 4A.17).

decision-making process. For example, three in five respondents (62 per cent) took early retirement despite regarding their financial package as being insufficient to sustain them in retirement. With regard to their labour market orientation, one in five (22 per cent) said they intended looking for part-time work after retiring; one in 14 respondents (7 per cent) would take on a full-time job and one in 20 respondents (5 per cent) would seek an opportunity for self-employment. Two out of three said they intended taking full retirement. When asked the reason for continuing employment, two-fifths (39 per cent) attributed this to the inadequacy of the financial package, a third wanted to be able to afford small luxuries and 18 per cent said they wanted to use their time productively.

There were important differences between salaried and hourly paid employees in the extent to which 'push' factors (the aspects of the job from which people are trying to escape) and 'pull' factors (the attractiveness of life in retirement) influenced early retirement decisions (Maule *et al.* 1996). While the retirement decision for hourly paid employees was dominated by 'push' factors – the negative aspects of their current job, such as shift work, as well as factors including ill health and fears over their future health – salaried employees were attracted by the positive potential offered by retirement opportunities, such as starting a new career or developing new hobbies or interests.

Research undertaken by Robertson *et al.* (2003) for the GO programme explored the experience of paid employment among people aged 50 to 75 and specifically on the relationship between participation in paid work and subsequent psychological wellbeing and life satisfaction – and the possible determinants of labour force participation at older ages. The study did not find statistically significant differences in wellbeing between their three categories of respondents (employed, unemployed, retired). *Employed* respondents reported the highest levels of subjective wellbeing (compared to those who were retired or unemployed). However, the highest levels of wellbeing in any category were found among those who were employed when over retirement age. This group was also shown to have the highest levels of life satisfaction. Those who were unemployed were found to have lowest levels of subjective wellbeing and life satisfaction. Wellbeing at older ages was found to be a function of personal choice as well as being dependent on the role held. Thus, wellbeing is not dependent just on whether one is employed or unemployed or retired but whether one wants to be. Individuals who want to work but are unable to do so may become frustrated; those who have to work because they need the income may be dissatisfied that they cannot retire.

Income and living standards

A key factor in QoL in older age is financial security. The 2002 ELSA study confirmed the strong correlation between socio-economic position (whether measured by income or wealth) and health. In 1979, 47 per cent of pensioner families were in the bottom fifth of the overall net income distribution (before housing costs); by 2001–2 this proportion had halved (Goodman *et al.* 2003). The Labour government is therefore going some way to meeting the Chancellor of the Exchequer's pledge 'to end pensioner poverty', made to the Labour Party Conference in September 2002. Microsimulation using the Institute for Fiscal Studies (IFS) tax and benefit model (Goodman *et al.* 2003) shows that government reforms aimed at pensioners have increased the incomes of single pensioners by 9 per cent, on average, and have increased those of pensioner couples by 5 per cent. The results also show that the poorest pensioners have gained most.

Despite the significant redistribution towards the poorest pensioners, poverty remains a long-term and intractable problem for large numbers of older people, which affects women in particular and is exacerbated for all as they get older; pensions lose value and savings diminish or disappear. In 2001–2, 11 per cent of pensioners were living on incomes below 50 per cent of median income (after housing costs); 22 per cent were living on incomes below 60 per cent (after housing costs). The latter is the measure of poverty used by the British Government's Social Exclusion Unit (DWP 2002), although it is about to adopt the measure of incomes *before* housing costs, which critics argue is less appropriate. The IFS acknowledges that the Labour government has latterly committed substantial resources to addressing poverty and that there has been some progress but casts doubt on whether this modest progress will be sustained:

> . . . despite large increases in benefits to pensioners, their incomes have only just managed to keep in line with, or move slightly ahead of, the median income enjoyed by the population as a whole, resulting in little change in relative poverty on most measures . . . when we set these changes in the context of a longer period of time, the fact that pensioners' incomes have kept in line with non-pensioner incomes during this period of rapid median income growth has been unusual, and pensioner incomes relative to non-pensioner incomes are higher than they have been at any time over the last 40 years. (Goodman *et al.* 2003: 21)

Younger age groups of older people, who are more likely to be in work, tend to receive more income from earnings. As people grow older they become more dependent on state and other pensions and their incomes are lower

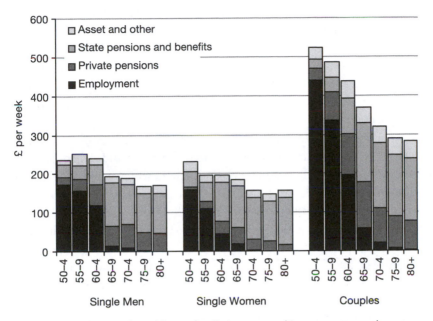

Figure 6.1 Mean total weekly net family income and income sources, by age
Source: Marmot *et al.* 2003.

(see Figure 6.1). This does not necessarily mean that income declines with age. Current 50 year olds may well receive different income levels when they reach older ages than those of the current generation of older people because of different lifetime characteristics, different policy environments and real economic growth over time (Marmot *et al.* 2003: 75). There is a key link between work life history and income in later life and, in some occupational groups, early retirement increases the risk of low income in old age (Walker 1981; Bardasi and Jenkins 2002). The ELSA data reveal that couples tend to have higher average levels of income than single people. Given that most single older people are women, this reinforces their greater vulnerability to poverty as they both live longer and, in general, have lower pensions because of their inferior participation in the labour market during their working lives. There are also inequalities in the distribution of income, wealth and non-pension wealth, according to age, gender and marital status. Older people, women and single people tend to be least well off according to each of these measures.

The contributory state retirement pension is received by 98 per cent of all pensioners. When it was introduced in 1948 it was intended that it should provide an adequate income for older people but it has proved insufficient for those without any other income or savings and significant numbers of older people have had to claim means-tested benefits. The value of the state pension has fallen by over 25 per cent in real terms since 1980 when the Conservative government introduced legislation that tied the increase to prices not earnings, thereby guaranteeing that the gap between pensioners and the working population would widen. Because of the low level of the state retirement pension approximately 2.5 million older people, over 30 per cent, receive a means-tested benefit (Help the Aged 2003). These include Minimum Income Guarantee (MIG), a social assistance benefit aimed at older people now replaced by a Pensioners' Tax Credit; housing benefit, which helps people with their rent; and council tax benefit, which is a subsidy towards local taxation. The maximum benefit entitlement (including all means-tested benefits) of a single pensioner under 75 in 2001–2 was £96 or 64 per cent of median income (after housing costs). For pensioner couples, it was £144.40 or 53 per cent (Goodman *et al.* 2003). Growing reliance by both Labour and Conservative governments on means-tested forms of assistance, rather than the increase in the state retirement pension argued for by many groups of older people and others (Townsend and Walker 1995; Ginn and Arber 1999), is perverse given the reluctance of many older people to claim such benefits. Non-takeup of benefits, which is higher among people over retirement age than among younger people, is a major cause of one-fifth of single pensioners and one in ten pensioner couples living on incomes below the poverty line. Government figures show that between 22 per cent and 36 per cent of pensioners who were entitled to MIG did not claim it in 1999–2000 (DWP 2001). One-third did not claim their council tax benefit entitlement and one in ten did not claim housing benefit (Goodman *et al.* 2003). A significant minority of pensioners are not entitled to these means-tested benefits, even though their actual income is below the necessary level, because they have savings above the capital limits that are imposed on eligibility. The Labour government has also introduced a number of payments in kind for older people to help with heating costs and the cost of the television licence, which must be paid by all television owners.

One major event to have an effect on the finances of older people is a partner's entry into a care home. One in ten older people in care homes are married and their partner is either living in the community or is also living in a residential setting. When the partner is living in the community the financial issues regarding state funding are complex. Only 1 per cent of people aged 65 to 74 live in care homes or long-stay hospitals but this figure rises to 25 per cent for people over 85 years old. In the over 80 age group there are approximately 2.3 women to every man (OPCS estimates reported in Jarvis *et al.* 1996: Table A.2). As well as living longer, women tend to marry men who are older than themselves and, because of this, outlive their husbands. They are, therefore, more likely to become widowed and stay in a long-stay care home (Hancock and Wright 1999).

There are three sources of state funding to help with the cost of institutional care, the social security system, Local Authority funding and the NHS (Hancock and Wright 1999). The first two are means tested so that people with income or capital above certain levels have to pay for their personal and social care needs in part or in full. Nursing care needs are met by the NHS. Local authorities set a baseline for care home fees that will be met (Hancock and Wright 1999) and there are considerable variations between different local authorities in England and Wales. Under the devolved powers given to Scotland, personal and social care as well as healthcare needs of older people have been paid for since 2002.

Conclusion

Although research on QoL in old age has a long history in the UK, it is only very recently that a systematic approach has taken shape and the perspectives of older people have been included. The GO programme has made a substantial contribution to knowledge on this subject (Walker and Hagan Hennessy 2004) and the ELSA provides an extensive new database but there are still large gaps particularly concerning the QoL and wellbeing of frail very elderly people.

Note

1. We are grateful to Kristiina Martimo for her help with this chapter and Chapter 11.

Part II

Quality of life in old age: participation, social support and subjective wellbeing

7

Germany: quality of life in old age II

Monika Reichert and Manuela Weidekamp-Maicher

Social relationships

In German gerontological research there are various approaches to measuring the quality of older people's social networks. 'Objective indicators' are the number of contact persons and the length of time spent with them, the number of common activities and the support function of social relationships. 'Subjective indicators' are the satisfaction and emotional wellbeing derived from them. In addition to the social support provided, the mere availability of certain social relationships is often linked with positive effects.

Epidemiological studies demonstrate the connection between good social integration and a high life expectancy. Older people who are extraverted and oriented to social contacts are not only more satisfied with their health but also demonstrate a higher degree of wellbeing (Lehr and Thomae 1987).

The quality of social relationships in old age must also be measured by subjective judgements by the older people themselves. One study concludes that the mere availability of various types of social relationships and contact frequency have *no* significant effect on subjective wellbeing (Schneider 1995). However, a high degree of perceived closeness and a high informational value *do* contribute significantly to subjective wellbeing (Buchmüller *et al.* 1996). The subjective assessment of network support is independent of the number of social relationships (Minnemann 1994a). Rather, the degree of adjustment of the network to the various needs of older people proved decisive for satisfaction. Furthermore, according to Minnemann (1992), satisfactory relationships in old age contribute to satisfaction with one's own ageing process.

Social relationships do not only influence QoL in old age in a positive sense; they can also become burdens. Negative experiences in dealing with other people have become a primary focus of research after it was demonstrated that they lead to a more sustained loss of wellbeing and mental health than is true, conversely, for positive social support. Thus it has been demonstrated that the dependence orientation of the social environment, which is reflected in overprotective behaviour, contributes to a long-term reduction in independent mastery and life satisfaction (Wahl 1991; Baltes 1995). The negative aspects of social relationships include the experience of excessive demands, loss of autonomy, lack of reciprocity, conflicts, use of force and neglect. Older people experience contact with others as burdensome if it is emotionally neutral or not meaningful.

Changes in social contacts can be attributed to changes in the goal and action orientation that is associated with ageing. Older people not only place great emphasis on emotional assistance and meaningful connections (Ferring and Filipp 1999), but also on the maintenance of 'threatened' values such as reciprocity, autonomy and self-sufficiency (Minnemann 1994a). Older people are often dependent on external help, due to the loss of function, but they have a great need to maintain self-sufficiency. This need – experiencing reciprocity and autonomy in relationships – exists mainly with those they are in very close contact with. Wellbeing in social relationships is maintained if older people can also experience their contact with other people as (self-)effective even in the face of functional impairment (Lang and Baltes 1997).

An essential database for analysing intergenerational relationships is the German Ageing Survey, which compiles information on the size and composition of social networks, the intensity of social contacts, and the benefits of social relationships (Kohli and Künemund 2000). This enables comparisons between objective and subjective measures. In the Bonn Gerontological Longitudinal Study (Lehr and Thomae 1987) and the Berlin Ageing Study (Mayer and Baltes 1996), the quality of social relationships was based on the number of contact persons, the role played in the relationship, the frequency of contacts, and the perceived closeness to the contact person (Wagner et al. 1996). Thus it is possible to make statements about connections between quantitative characteristics of social networks and subjective evaluations.

Loneliness and quality of life

The significance of private social relationships in old age is increasing due to a gradual decrease in integration in formal institutions such as employment.

Therefore, having solid social contacts and an active lifestyle in old age is very significant for good health, life satisfaction and QoL (Lehr and Minnemann 1987; Lehr 1994). For example, the significance of social contacts for subjective wellbeing in older people is illustrated by the close connection between the scope of social activities and mood (Tesch-Römer 1998). Social isolation and loneliness are 'antitheses' of social activity.

Living alone and being alone can be perceived as positive or negative and do not mean, *per se*, loneliness or isolation. Social isolation describes a lack of social relationships. The presence of very few social contacts of a very short duration is frequently used as an indicator of social isolation. Weiss (1982, cited in Tesch-Römer 2000) distinguished between 'social' and 'emotional' isolation. Social isolation refers to the absence of a social network or quantitative deficiencies in a network, whereas emotional isolation refers to the lack of a confidant; this type of isolation seems to be especially significant in giving rise to loneliness (Wagner *et al.* 1996; Smith and Baltes 1996; Tesch-Römer 2000). Loneliness arises because of an imbalance between one's own social needs and the actual situation in which those needs are supposed to be met. People compare the quality, the number and role variability of their social relationships with the desires they have with respect to these relationships. If the perceived network of one's own expectations is different, feelings of loneliness or isolation are the result (Tesch-Römer 2000). Both social and emotional loneliness are positively related to age (Mayer and Baltes 1996; Wagner *et al.* 1996). The connection between age and emotional loneliness is greater than the connection between age and social loneliness, and perceived deficiencies in confidant relationships are the best predictor of emotional loneliness. Both types of loneliness are easier to predict using subjective measures of satisfaction than by the size of the networks. Age and gender (women feel lonelier than men, and very old people feel more lonely than young-old ones) as well as satisfaction with family and friends explain most of the variance of emotional loneliness. Thus Smith and Baltes (1996) conclude that loneliness is is the combination of being alone with the feeling of emotional loneliness.

Most older people are more firmly rooted in social contexts with relatives and family than is generally believed (Lehr and Minnemann 1987; Wagner *et al.* 1996; Kohli and Szydlik 2000). However, this applies especially to young-old people (Töpfer *et al.* 1998). Studies looking at the situation of the very old indicate that social isolation is more probable than among younger cohorts (Lehr and Minnemann 1987; Wagner *et al.* 1996). Increasing

161

'singularization' in old age corresponds with a rise in feelings of loneliness. About one-third of those aged 60 and over indicate they sometimes or often experience feelings of loneliness (Federal Statistical Office 1997, cited by Tesch-Römer 2000).

In 2000, 37 per cent of all one-person households belonged to older people (over 65), and 77 per cent of them were widowed (Federal Statistical Office 2000). While one-third of men over 80 years of age live in one-person households, for women it is around 70 per cent. Although living alone and being alone are not in themselves sufficient conditions for loneliness they are among its risk factors. 75 per cent of those saying they are lonely live by themselves, and only 5 per cent live in three-person or multiple-person households (Dannenbeck 1995). With increasing age, the amount of time spent alone increases: from an average of about 12 hours/day in middle age (ages 35 to 44) to about 15 hours/day for those 60 to 64 and 17 hours/day for those over 70 (Küster 1998).

Social isolation is accompanied by reduced subjective wellbeing (Adler et al. 2000). In addition to social isolation, the type and quality of older people's social networks are also responsible for whether they feel lonely. In the Berlin Ageing Study, only 3 per cent of all participants indicated 'no-one' as their entire social network. Those aged 70 to 84 years indicated significantly more people in their social network than those aged 85 and over. Those aged 85 and over said they had no confidants in the outermost circles of their network. The absolute size of the social network is significant: older people describe themselves as lonely especially if they have either very small or relatively large networks; a medium-sized network apparently offers the best protection against loneliness (Minnemann 1994b).

The death of one's life partner is often accompanied by loneliness or 'forced isolation' (Dannenbeck 1995). Thus, almost 50 per cent of all those interviewed who indicated they were lonely were widowed and 17 per cent were divorced. Other significant relationships include children: childlessness is an important risk factor for loneliness in old age. A connection is demonstrated between not being lonely and having children (Wagner et al. 1996). The fact of having a child plays an important role, but no additional protection against social isolation in old age is afforded by a greater number of children.

The services and functions provided by a social network are also relevant for the development of loneliness; a lack of emotional support is more significant than a lack of instrumental help (Wagner et al. 1996). When recording and predicting subjective wellbeing, the existence of at least one close confidant is a better predictor than objectively measurable factors (Thomae 1994). In the Berlin Ageing Study, however, almost 50 per cent of those interviewed indicated they had no confidants of this type (Wagner *et al.* 1996). Losses within the circle of closest confidents were among the greatest risks of advanced age (Marbach 2001). Along with the characteristics of social networks, the health of a person is an independent risk factor for loneliness. Older people subject to health-related limitations, particularly loss of mobility, experience loneliness more often than older people without them (Wagner *et al.* 1996).

Grandparenting

The role of grandparents has been emphasized recently in German research, in particular with regard to the exchange of support within the family, which highlights the special significance of grandparents as *givers* of financial support to younger family members (Kohli and Künemund 2001). But the role of today's grandparents is not clearly defined and can range from grandparents going completely unnoticed to their exercising long-term obligations and tasks.

Even though older people show a high degree of willingness to care for (potential) grandchildren (84 per cent of those aged 40 to 59), the experience of grandparenting depends on several factors. For example, the relationships between grandparents and grandchildren differ between younger and older grandparents. Grandparenting is perceived as an enriching experience if it falls in the period of young old age. Another factor that determines differences in the interactions between grandparents and grandchildren is the gender of both partners (Künemund 1997). While grandfathers attempt to have an influence on their grandchildren primarily in an instrumental manner, with suggestions and financial support, the relationships of grandmothers to their grandchildren are characterized mostly by emotional aspects. In looking after their grandchildren, grandmothers often take on caring tasks and experience this relationship as more satisfying than do grandfathers (Sticker 1987). Frequency of contact between grandparents and grandchildren is determined, along with geographical distance between the two residences, by the age of both the grandparents and the grandchildren. The contacts become less frequent the older the grandchildren become: two-fifths of grandparents have daily contact with grandchildren when they are toddlers (Sticker 1987). Whereas grandparents whose grandchildren have reached the age of young adults often do not see each other more fre-quently than once every few months. Those with one grandchild are much more involved than 'experienced' grandparents with multiple grandchildren. With the increasing age of grandchildren, not only the contact behaviour changes but also the function of the grandparents (Kohli and Künemund 2001). While grand-parents of grandchildren of toddler and pre-school age mostly assume caring responsibilities, as the grandchildren grow older other functions such as emotional affection and conveying knowledge become more significant. The role of grandparents as models decreases as the age of the grandchildren increases and the relationship also seems to become less intense.

The relationship between grandparents and grandchildren is considered prototypical of those between old and young people. With regard to the signif-icance of the quality of this relationship, the question has been raised of whether older people need relationships with young people and, if so, how these relationships can increase QoL? Lang and Baltes (1997) point out that the relationship to grandchildren can be seen in the context of the develop-mental tasks of old age. In grandparenting, older people primarily address their need for generativity (see below).

Active ageing and participation

In the past 20 years, research on activity in old age has indicated that, by itself, it does not contribute to life satisfaction; rather, it is the congruity between an individual lifestyle and an activity repertoire of skills, interests and values. Nevertheless physical and mental activities represent an important basis for healthy ageing. They are also associated with less institutionalization, better physical and mental health, greater longevity and general wellbeing (Lehr and Thomae 1987; Helmchen *et al.* 1996). Research indicates an important connection between physical activity, physical and mental health, and general wellbeing (Helmchen *et al.* 1996; Borchelt *et al.* 1996). Physical activity also has a positive influence on functional health (the activities of daily living). In older people, physical activity also generates positive effects on body image and self-confidence and contributes to a better self assessment. Physical activity is able to reduce stress (Fuchs *et al.* 1994) and depression (Hautzinger and Kleine 1995). The SIMA study found that physical activity significantly improves cognitive performance in old age and a combined memory and psychomotor training programme thus resulted in improved cognitive performance (Oswald *et al.* 1998).

Both social and cognitive activities also make an essential contribution to the wellbeing of older people. Social activities often strengthen long-term existing roles in the life of an older person and preserve the continuity of social identity. The Berlin Ageing Study (Smith *et al.* 1996; Wagner *et al.* 1996) and studies on life satisfaction and wellbeing indicate that satisfaction with partners and family represents one of the most important life goals (Hauser *et al.* 1996).

Several recent studies focus on the significance of cognitive activity for successful ageing (Helmchen *et al.* 1996; Oswald *et al.* 1998; Kliegel *et al.* 2001). They show that people who had been in jobs with few cognitive demands demonstrated noticeable loss in memory performance, whereas those who constantly took on new responsibilities and tasks demonstrated better cognitive status. Cognitive activities such as a memory training programme contribute to improvements in cognitive performance, more independence and wellbeing, even in advanced old age. The 'Rules for healthy ageing' emphasize an active lifestyle and the significance of physical, mental and social activity for wellbeing in old age (Kruse and Schmitt 1998).

Leisure

When assessing leisure activities, activity as such does not correlate with life satisfaction but rather with the subjective feeling of social affirmation or social integration. A low level of activity can be correlated positively with life satisfaction if it ensures sufficient feelings of social integration and self-fulfilment. Leisure activities can promote both social integration and individual autonomy. A positive concept of leisure in old age is based on notions of the potential of old age and generativity. The potential of old age means the unused resources and competencies for a fulfilling, satisfying and meaningful life in old age. Generativity is the notion of a stronger participation in the life of later generations as well as the transfer of responsibility in order to maintain societal and cultural values. Leisure activities also contribute to a new role identity by offering an opportunity to compensate for past work roles.

Various time-use analyses indicate that those who are no longer working have on average 6.5 hours of leisure time available per day (Küster 1998). According to Baltes *et al.* (1996b), leisure activities take up 34 per cent of waking time of 70- to 84-year-olds, and 42 per cent of waking time of those aged 85 and over. The increase in time older people can spend as they wish, however, is related to a decrease in activity level, which means that with greater age the participation in leisure activities decreases. The relationship between old age and activity level is moderated by other factors such as social class and educational level and, in particular, interest in cultural events, participation in continuing education programmes, and volunteer work (Mayer and

Baltes 1996; Kohli and Künemund 1997). This is also confirmed by Kolland (1996): if educational attainment is controlled for, age loses its significant influence on cultural behaviour.

Even though improved economic conditions mean that older people have many different opportunities for spending time and the increase in free time invites them to do so, health concerns in old age limit the existing scope of action. The result of the ensuing restrictions in the activity radius is that certain kinds of lifestyle or habitual ways of spending leisure time can no longer be maintained because a certain competency in basic functions of daily life is a necessary condition for performing leisure activities (Baltes *et al.* 1996b). This includes activities of daily living as well as cognitive competencies. If the prospects for self-structuring diminish, externally imposed structuring must become more important. Even competencies that are not necessarily related to individual ability can and should be protected by corresponding social intervention and technical aids or services.

Volunteering

One possibility for experiencing meaning in old age is provided by voluntary work. Psychological gerontology refers to such involvement in terms of 'productive ageing', which opens up new opportunities for maintaining an independent lifestyle and the transferrence of experience and mutual support among older people (Von Rosenbladt 2000). Older people who are involved in volunteering can tap into social networks and thus expand the scope of their activities.

The most commonly expressed motives for undertaking voluntary work among 60-year-olds are: 'to help other people' (62 per cent), 'to be accepted as you are' (58 per cent), 'to feel needed' (56 per cent), and 'to have fun with people your own age' (52 per cent) (Ueltzhöffer 1999). In deciding to become involved in voluntary work, especially among the young old, 'self-related' motives are more important than 'self-less' ones. This points to the specific needs of older people for new forms of participation that, at the same time, are connected with high expectations in terms of the content, variety and diversity. The opportunities for taking initiative and for self-determination play a major role (BMFSFJ 2001a).

The potential of older people as volunteers is significantly greater than their actual involvement. Voluntary activity was quantified in 1996: 22 per cent for ages 40 to 54, 13 per cent for the 55 to 69 group, and 7 per cent for ages 70 to 85 (Kohli and Künemund 1997). Official figures confirm these findings and also show that voluntary involvement is higher in younger age groups than in old age: the percentage of volunteers in the groups aged 14 to 24 and 25 to 59 was 37 per cent and among those aged 60 years and over it was 26 per cent (BMFSFJ 2001a). The reason for relatively low participation in voluntary work among older people is not disinterest but a lack of information on opportunities for involvement. The fear of not being taken seriously as a volunteer as well as the assumption that one is too old to carry out voluntary activity are also reasons for low levels of such participation (BMFSFJ 2001a). The decline in voluntary work in old age is also often associated with a worsening state of health. Thus, even with highly active older people, health is an essential reason for a decline in activity (Künemund 2000b). The involvement of older people in special programmes aimed at them is unexpectedly low and recent research indicates that such programmes should be designed across age groups due to a negative societal image of older people.

Nursing care and support systems

The significance of public support arrangements for QoL in old age is important not only because of a continuing decline in family assistance, but also from the perspectives of raising the quality of nursing care and emphasizing its contribution to wellbeing in old age. The focus in research on long-term care in Germany was initially concentrated on defining and recording objective indicators because it was assumed that they contribute the most to QoL. The dimensions of subjective QoL, such as satisfaction and emotional wellbeing, have only recently become a focus of research.

The legal guidelines on long-term care insurance determine the limits within which nursing care and assistance can be offered and performed. They also determine which services are rendered so that they both indirectly and directly influence the QoL of older people in need of care. The nursing-care system in Germany, which has undergone major changes since the introduction of the law on long-term care insurance (Social Statutes XI – SGB XI),[1] makes various forms of support available to older people. Depending on the degree of impairment, the availability of other help, or personal preferences, older people can select between inpatient nursing care (residential long-term institutions), daily care, or outpatient care. For nursing-care insurance to cover these costs, however, those involved must demonstrate a considerable degree of disability in carrying out normal activities of daily life.

Ensuring the best possible QoL is not one of the explicit goals of statutory nursing-care insurance. Quality is only oriented to objectifiable features of nursing care (Social Statutes XI – SGB XI). For a long time this view dominated the public and scientific debates, until deficiencies in the law, and especially disparities in its implementation, put the focus on additional quality features of nursing care and other evaluation criteria. In future, orientation to the needs and desires of the users of nursing care should be more prominent.

Ensuring the quality of nursing care

A high level of quality in caring for dependent people has only been considered an important policy goal since the introduction of nursing-care insurance. Inpatient and outpatient facilities are obliged by law to demonstrate quality assurance procedures. This demand was followed by a controversial debate about suitable measures for ensuring the quality of nursing-care services. The original emphasis in guaranteeing high quality nursing care was on the development of quality standards and on the search for quality criteria for other factors such as architectural standards or the qualifications of nursing staff. Research also focused on the development of methods and instruments of quality assurance (Görres 1999), including the Geriatric Assessment Task Force (AGAST 1995) in geriatrics and the Resident Assessment Instrument (RAI) in long-term care (Gilgen and Garms-Homolóva 1995). However, the essential problems in using such instruments for quality assurance continue to exist, for example, in determining the criteria and standards for assessing quality. Moreover, research on the specific contributions of different forms of care in improving QoL in old age has not been carried out.

The user perspective

In the search for suitable criteria for evaluating nursing care the issue of patient satisfaction has taken on an increasingly central role in research. Such studies focus not only on the expectations that older people have in terms of facilities and services but also on satisfaction with nursing services. Although the current state of research is unsatisfactory with regard to the preferences of potential and current users of nursing services – in particular, there is a lack of studies that include the subjective wellbeing of older people – several studies have been conducted. They report positive evaluations of the quality of care, in particular of outpatient care provided by nursing-care insurance, which is assessed as 'very satisfactory' or as 'overall satisfactory' (Becker et al. 1998; Blinkert and Klie 1999). The high degree of satisfaction with the in-home care situation of older people corresponds directly with their level of expectation and the alternative of inpatient care. Because older people fear the risk of nursing-home care, the overall assessment is always positive even if there are criticisms of the care (Becker *et al.* 1998).

If they express criticism, older users are dissatisfied mainly with the organization of outpatient services. Fault is found in particular with telephone accessibility and hours of operation, which are not geared to their daily rhythm but to organizational requirements (Becker *et al.* 1998). Older service users until now have been very reluctant to take advantage of services that exceed the minimum level of assistance guaranteed by nursing-care insurance, especially when these services must be paid for privately (Evers and Rauch 1998). Changes in personnel are also experienced as stressful. Patients experience their personal living space as the workplace of a large number of staff where they are robbed of their personal identity. Frequent changes in personnel act as a hindrance in establishing stable nursing relationships, thus reducing the perceived QoL, and also contribute to disorientation among those suffering from dementia. The desire for a long-term confidant with whom a relationship of trust can be established has the highest priority for older people. Other subjective quality criteria include a circle of helpers that is as small and manageable as possible, reliability, transparency, better time management, friendliness and empathy (Schaeffer 1999). The inclusion of need and user preferences as criteria for organizing care, however, generally clashes with the way the services traditionally work and are organized. A lack of flexibly, tight organizational restrictions in terms of time and money and an orientation to the average person in need of care are factors that often prove to be impediments to change.

Furthermore, there are differences in QoL evaluation criteria between patients and professionals. While residents of long-term care institutions or users of outpatient services define their QoL primarily in terms of wellbeing, their family members and nursing staff see it in terms of the quality of the nursing. Similarly in the evaluation of nursing services: experts are oriented to standards with the highest possible quality of nursing but users emphasize social and communicative elements of the nursing (Sowarka 2000). Older users attribute greater importance not to the expertise of the nursing staff but to the way the staff treat them.

In terms of planned improvements in QoL in nursing homes it is important to include the perspectives of the very old because they are the ones who use the services. In nursing homes, 67 per cent of all residents are over 80 years of age. Among the users of in-home services those aged 85 to 90 make up the largest group (19.4 per cent), followed by the 80 to 85 year olds (13.7 per cent). Women are the largest group receiving both inpatient and outpatient care (BMFSFJ 2001a). User-oriented care should therefore consider the age and gender of older people when surveying preferences and needs. Nursing care insurance attempted to strengthen the position of older users but services are still not being managed in accordance with their needs. The challenge of consulting those suffering from dementia, who are not in a position to communicate their own needs, has not been faced.

Deficiencies in care insurance law

In addition to the lack of user orientation, the care insurance law promotes a deficiency model of ageing. For example, highest priority is given by the law to rehabilitation but this is not reflected in the provision of care. As each improvement in the health of the patient is necessarily accompanied by reductions in services, there is no motivation to follow the rehabilitation approach. Nursing-care services are thus determined by financial criteria and not by their relevance to the user. Nursing that is oriented to the deficiency model is reduced to body-related aspects. This not only acts as an impediment to holistic nursing but also prescribes a narrow view of nursing that reduces it to technical activities and excludes the communicative, psychosocial and educational competencies of older people.

The number who are entitled to care is considerable but not all of those in need are able to enjoy the services provided by nursing-care insurance and an expansion of services is also needed. People with minor health-related restrictions are excluded from these services. This includes older people who would stand to benefit the most from proactive, preventive forms of care. The law is deficient with regard to the care of those who deviate from the physical criteria for defining need, which primarily affects people with dementia and other psychiatric illnesses. The practice of cost effectiveness is not tailored to the staff-intensive care of those suffering from dementia with the result that the quality of nursing care for older people with dementia is substandard.

The introduction of nursing-care insurance was accompanied by a large expansion of the community sector. Older users have been overwhelmed by the new access channels and confusing array of services. However, there is a lack of special services that go beyond the needs of the average user. Those older people who have no relatives are dependent on consulting services or consumer protection services to help them make the right choice.

Improvements can be expected in the future following the new Nursing Quality Assurance Act and amendment to the Act on Residential Accommodation. Nursing homes will be required to improve internal quality assurance. Each nursing service must implement and continue to develop a comprehensive, internal quality assurance programme. Quality must be demonstrated by independent experts or organizations. In addition to better consulting services, lists that compare local services and prices will provide more competition and increase the transparency of services for the insured.

The new Act on Residential Accommodation is aimed at improving the legal situation of residents. Home agreements will all have the same form in order to allow comparisons with other facilities. Opportunities for involving residents in the process of nursing will be improved as will other creative opportunities in the nursing home. The home advisory committee (consisting of representatives of the residents and their relatives or confidantes) will play an essential role in internal decisions. It will also be integrated into the process of quality assurance and evaluation.

The goal of both laws is to strengthen the position of the users and to create greater transparency in the nursing-care market. Older people in need of care will have more opportunities for making decisions and becoming involved. More advice on their rights will allow those customers who are in need of special protection to be included in the process of nursing care. In this way the conditions will be created to include subjective criteria of QoL in the process of nursing.

Life satisfaction and subjective wellbeing

Findings on the relationship between old age and subjective wellbeing are inconsistent (Mayring 1987; BMFSFJ 2002a). Some studies show that the level of subjective wellbeing increases with age whereas others indicate the opposite. For example, one study (BMFSFJ 2002a) shows that very elderly people generally experience a high level of wellbeing in spite of their losses and limitations: 87 per cent of those over 70 years of age in West Germany and 82 per cent of East Germans of the same age felt very or fairly happy. In comparison with the whole population, however, older people more frequently reported that they were unhappy. In West Germany there were 13 per cent in the oldest age group and 19 per cent in East Germany (Noll and Schöb 2001, cited in BMFSFJ 2002a: 92).

The lack of consistency in findings suggests that the different components of subjective wellbeing should be recorded separately, as in the Welfare Survey

(WS). The different living conditions in West and East Germany also mean that it is necessary to record QoL separately. Table 7.1 shows the satisfaction of older people in various areas of life.

Table 7.1 Satisfaction with specific living conditions in late adulthood and old age

Satisfaction with specific domains of life (on average)[1]	Adults between the ages of 55 and 69		Older people aged 70 and over	
	West Germany	East Germany	West Germany	East Germany
Standard of living	7.5	7.0	8.0	7.5
Health	6.7	6.3	6.3	5.9
Housing conditions	8.6	7.9	8.9	8.2
Residential environment	8.3	7.7	8.7	7.9
Family life	8.8	8.8	8.9	9.1
Opportunities for political participation	6.0	5.7	6.0	5.2
Leisure time	8.1	7.7	8.4	7.9

Note
1. In the Welfare Survey, satisfaction with specific domains of life is measured by using 11-point Likert-scales (from 0 = 'very dissatisfied' to 10 = 'very satisfied').
Source: Noll and Schöb (2002).

Table 7.2 shows global measures of wellbeing based on the last WS (1998).

The relationship between objective living conditions and subjective evaluations was examined in the comprehensive Berlin Ageing Study, as was general subjective wellbeing (Smith *et al.* 1996). The results provide a positive picture of wellbeing in old age, even if there are considerable differences in individual experience (Staudinger *et al.* 1996). The majority of those surveyed aged 70 to 103 (63 per cent) indicated they were satisfied with life in the past and present and had relatively few concerns as they looked to the future (Smith *et al.* 1996). The analyses confirm that objective living conditions cannot by themselves predict overall wellbeing. Component-specific evaluations also need to be considered. Only gender and residental status had a direct effect upon wellbeing. Women expressed less life satisfaction than men, and nursing home residents indicated a lower level of subjective wellbeing than people who lived in their own homes. The strongest predictors of subjective wellbeing were the subjective evaluations of the various domains of life.

Table 7.2 Satisfaction with the general life situation, happiness and anomie symptoms in late adulthood and old age

Overall measures of wellbeing:	Adults between the ages of 55 and 69		Older people aged 70 and over	
	West Germany	East Germany	West Germany	East Germany
happiness[1] (%)				
(I am) very happy	18	17	16	10
quite happy	72	72	71	72
quite unhappy	10	11	13	17
very unhappy	0	–	0	2
life satisfaction[2]				
	7.9	7.4	7.7	7.6
anomie symptoms[1] (%)				
today's difficulties cannot be changed	69	86	84	87
contemporary life has become complicated	14	29	23	38
no future prospects	38	43	39	48

Notes
1. The measures of happiness and anomie symptoms are expressed as a percentage of all persons asked in the survey who agreed to the statement 'it is absolutely right' and 'it is quite right'.
2. Overall satisfaction with life is measured by using 11-point Likert-scales (from 0 = 'very dissatisfied' to 10 = 'very satisfied'). The measures show the general life satisfaction on average.

In terms of the emotional component of subjective wellbeing, positive affects become less frequent from young adulthood and on into very old age, while the level of negative affect remains relatively stable (Ferring and Filipp 1997a). Even though very old people have positive emotions more frequently than negative ones, the Berlin Ageing Study showed that with increasing age there is a decrease in positive emotions and in anticipated future life satisfaction (Staudinger *et al.* 1996). It was not possible to determine any differences in age groups in terms of current life satisfaction and overall wellbeing. At the same time, the authors emphasize the limits imposed by the risk of infirmity, functional loss and poor health among very old people (85 and over).

The paradox of life satisfaction in old age

Cross-sectional surveys of wellbeing among different age groups often showed that older people, despite health and other problems, have higher satisfaction levels than younger age groups. This fact has often been the subject of empirical studies (Staudinger and Freund 1998; Staudinger 2000). Research on coping has shown that there are many mental adaptation strategies responsible for protecting the integrity of subjective wellbeing of older people (Brandstädter and Greve 1992). This high degree of resilience in old and very old people is a significant potential of old age (Staudinger and Greve 2001). Nonetheless, this high level of adaptability is also a problem in planning policy interventions. Older people seldom express dissatisfaction with their life situation so there is a danger that, despite an 'objective' need to do so, they will not take advantage of these opportunities or that opportunities will not be created (Naegele 1998). At least one qualitative study by Mayring (1991) has shown that wellbeing in youth and old age is based on different factors. Among younger people wellbeing tends to be based more on current, situation-specific and intensive feelings – while in old age it is based more on overall happiness and good living conditions.

Wellbeing does not seem to follow a constant pattern over the life course. Distinguishing between long-term and current subjective wellbeing has been shown to be useful (Mayring 1991). Various studies point out that long-term wellbeing demonstrates a high level of constancy over the lifecourse. In psychological gerontology this is explained by the stability of personality features and coping strategies (Staudinger and Greve 2001). Thus coping strategies represent an essential mechanism for safeguarding wellbeing (Brandstädter and Greve 1992). In the case of irreversible losses, palliative coping strategies – for example, setting new standards in self-evaluation, devaluation of no longer attainable life goals, or the positive reinterpretation of situations – become more important. As it becomes more probable that someone will experience irreversible losses in old age, greater significance is attached to adaptive coping. Adjustment to a situation that is seen as being unchangeable contributes to maintaining subjective wellbeing among older people.

Future research priorities

(Re)Conceptualization of quality of life in old age

Recording QoL in old age is problematic for two reasons: different definitions of the concept across disciplines and the absence of theory. These problems make it difficult to measure the construct and compare the results from different studies.

In terms of the conceptualization of the term 'quality of life in old age', there are several matters that are unresolved. One of them concerns the definition of individual dimensions as well as their relative weighting. Here there is a need for further theoretical considerations as well as empirical research that inquires into the criteria of QoL, in particular from the perspective of older people. The dimension of goal congruence proposed by Mayring (1987) could prove to be instructive in terms of the conceptualization of individual components of subjective QoL, chiefly life satisfaction. This dimension could help not only to record significant life goals and needs in old age but also explain the changes they undergo (cf. Ferring and Filipp 1997a).

Health

Health is considered to be one of the central issues in old age (Dittmann-Kohli 1995) and subjective health has also become one of the best predictors of subjective wellbeing in later life. However, there is a lack of suitable information about the criteria older people themselves use to estimate and evaluate their health. Future research should therefore concentrate more on the recording of individual evaluations or the subjective health theories of older people. Knowledge of changes of cognitive status in the fourth age is also deficient. In future increasing explanatory value is likely to be given to cognitive changes at the end of the lifespan with regard to heterogeneity in indicators of health, psychological ability and the life context. Future research should therefore concentrate on explaining dissimilarities in the ageing process. Knowledge about these processes can contribute to increasing the number of years with the highest possible QoL (Dinkel 1999).

Research on QoL and dementia will probably become more significant. Cognitive loss is considered to pose the greatest danger for a total loss of QoL in old age. Studies on the QoL of those suffering from dementia are rare. An example is the study by Meier (1995, cited in BMFSFJ 2002a: 50ff), which found that people suffering from dementia emphasize dimensions different from those that are represented in traditional standardized QoL scales. For this reason it is necessary to construct appropriate instruments for recording subjective wellbeing of those affected, which are based on self-reported data.

Intervention research to increase quality of life

In Germany there is a general lack of applied research on improving QoL among the very elderly. In intervention research there is a lack of studies on the effectiveness of rehabilitation, of psychosocial interventions with people suffering from dementia or on the evaluation of interventions with caring relatives. Longitudinal studies of larger samples are especially necessary. The relatively poor research situation with respect to evaluations of different interventions with the very elderly can be attributed to the deficient state of knowledge about the very elderly in general. Studies in this area are still rare in Germany, as confirmed by the commission of the federal government's Fourth Ageing Report. From 1994 to 2004 only 3.5 per cent of the articles published in German gerontological journals dealt with advanced age, and of the 190 gerontological research groups in Germany a mere 10 per cent concentrated on advanced old age (BMFSFJ 2002a: 41). The majority of large German panel studies on ageing deal only with questions about the transition from middle age to the third age.

Living conditions

The search for the criteria for good living conditions in the fourth age is a special challenge for research on QoL. Another concerns the safeguarding of the QoL for people suffering from dementia. The opportunities and limitations of technological innovations to allow this group to live in a private household should also be topics of research. The contribution of technology is related to features of the equipment and furnishings which enable older people to have an independent lifestyle in spite of health problems. The question must also be raised about how technological innovations can contribute to improving the safety of the living situation. Research should examine subjective criteria for the acceptance of technology and the technical competencies of older people.

Social relationships

The process of private network building is currently undergoing comprehensive change. This is already evident in the restructuring of makeup and assignment of tasks within the networks of older people. For example, professional helpers are taking on more and more responsibilities that until now were borne by informal, usually family based help networks. Research should focus on the reconstitution of support arrangements, the allocation of responsibilities within the support networks, as well as how this change will affect the wellbeing of older people.

The pattern of future care arrangements for older people should be researched. Although the Ageing Study data do not forecast any serious quantitative collapses in family structures within the next 30 years (Kohli and Szydlik 2000), this should not hide the fact that families in the future, for reasons of labour mobility and changed notions of solidarity, will not be able to take on all of the care responsibilities for older people. Moreover, there will be a growing minority of older people in the future who will have no family support or only limited family support.

Therefore, the question must be raised whether new functional roles between informal and formal networks will become necessary in the future and, if so, what the effects will be on QoL. In particular, for those older people who have insufficient resources, or no resources, professional resources of a kind unknown to date will have to play a compensatory role.

Work, leisure and participation

There are two important perspectives here. The first is related to improving opportunities for managing time during the retirement years. Tasks must be found that are significant for society and at the same time can contribute to personal meaning. Knowledge is required about the features of voluntary work that can increase subjective wellbeing in old age. The second perspective is the question about possibilities for managing the time of older, physically handicapped persons. Older people who live in their own homes and who cannot leave them due to mobility restrictions are subject to the risks of social isolation and loneliness. Designing compensatory activities to replace leisure activities that can no longer be performed and the possibilities for maintaining social contacts, should therefore become a central focus of research.

Ethnic minorities

There is little data on QoL among older migrants. On the basis of currently available information only a few statements can be made about the objective QoL of these groups and only conjectures about the subjective wellbeing of older foreigners living in Germany. The cause of this deficit is the common exclusion of these groups from the large panel surveys. A survey of subjective indicators of life satisfaction among older migrants would be of interest.

Conclusion

German-language studies indicate that the significance of private social relationships in old age is increasing due to the gradual reduction in integration into formal structures such as employment. Moreover, increasing 'singularization' in old age corresponds with a rising risk of social isolation and feelings of loneliness. Satisfaction with life and subjective wellbeing of older people, especially for those who live alone and are not in touch with younger generations, will probably depend more on the degree to which society creates new opportunities to build up individually shaped social networks. German research on QoL and subjective wellbeing in old age point out that age-related losses of QoL are mostly due to social losses – social relationships, social roles, satisfaction with ones own leisure time, activities and mobility – rather than losses of material conditions and dissatisfaction with income. While the long-standing protection of material security for the older generations is clearly reflected in the high level of satisfaction with material and financial living conditions, the issue of how to improve the quality of social life will become a challenge for future cohorts of older people.

Note

1. Translator's note: SGB = Sozialgesetzbuch (Code of Social Law).

8

Italy: quality of life in old age II

Francesca Polverini and Giovanni Lamura

Introduction

Chapter 3 emphasized the fundamental influence exerted by the family on the quality of life (QoL) of older people in Italy. Despite the dramatic demographic changes that have occurred in the last few decades in Italy the family (often to be understood as an extended family, that is a network of households linked by kinship) still remains the main source of support for many older people, both from the point of view of social contacts and for the provision of care needs in case of dependency, a fact that is confirmed by the low rate of older people living in institutions (Renzi *et al.* 1995; Pace 1996; Tomassini 2004).

The debate on the central role of the family in Italian social life has been rather lively, especially in the past – for example, Banfield (1976) referred to the 'amoral familism' of the rural society in Southern Italy in the 1950s – but this factor is still a basic element in the QoL of older people in Italy (Presidenza del Consiglio dei Ministri 2000).

Family and support networks

On analysing the family structure of older people in Italy in comparison with those prevailing in other European countries, one of the most striking aspects is the relatively low percentage of older people living alone (Table 1.3). The percentage of older persons living with other family members is also higher in Italy than in other countries.

The gap between Italy and northern EU countries is wide, but the data in Table 8.1 show that, since the early 1980s, the number of older people living alone has almost doubled.

Table 8.1 Changes in living arrangements for families with at least one older member, 1981–98 (as a percentage of all families)

	1981	1991	1998
Older person living alone	7.8	11.6	13.2
Household with older members only	14.8	19.2	23.0
Other kinds of household with older people only	7.0	7.5	9.8

Source: De Vincenti and Rodano (2001).

There is also a strong gender division: older men's family experience is mainly one shared with their spouses (and in younger age groups with their children), older women's experience, especially above 75, is to a large extent solitary (Table 8.2). This is explained by women's greater longevity and the traditionally younger age of women at marriage, which contributes to the large number of over 65-year-old widows (49 per cent, against 12 per cent of men), in contrast with a prevalence of married men in the same age group (81 per cent against 41 per cent of women).

At the same time, as has been observed in other countries (Walter 1999), more and more older people wish to have regular contact with their children and grandchildren but, at the same time, to live in a separate household. This desire for 'intimacy at a distance' reflects the growing number of older people with a sense of respect for individual privacy but who do not want to renounce the possibility of continuous contact and reciprocal help among relatives, and appreciate the physical proximity of their households (Florea 1994).

This is also linked to the growing difficulty experienced by many Italian families in providing the necessary care to their most elderly members (Lamura *et al.* 2001). This trend – which is partly a consequence of the increasing

Table 8.2 Older population by family type and gender (%)

	Males			Females		
	60–4	65–74	Over 75	60–4	65–74	Over 75
Couple with children	52.2	28.3	11.8	32.2	12.4	2.8
Couple without children	33.0	53.2	59.4	36.4	41.2	18.1
Living alone	6.9	8.8	15.8	13.3	6.9	44.7
Other family types	7.9	9.7	13.0	18.1	19.5	34.4

Source: ISTAT (2001a).

participation in the labour market of the adult women's generations (OECD 1996; Lamura *et al.* 1999a) – affects the QoL both of the older people who receive care and the family caregivers, who are increasingly forced to resort to the help of foreign immigrants as cohabiting helpers (Socci *et al.* 2001, 2003) or, more rarely, to look for support measures such as respite services and carers' leave (Lamura *et al.* 1999b; Pellegrino 2000; Melchiorre *et al.* 2001).

When focusing on three main categories of family relationships – spouse, children and grandchildren – it should be kept in mind that family relationships involve a whole series of different members of the extended kin network, as shown by the fact that 30 per cent of the over-65s say that they can rely, in case of need, on the help of relatives different from these three categories, such as for instance nieces and nephews (37 per cent), brothers- and sisters-in-law (30 per cent), cousins (28 per cent) and sons- and daughters-in-law (20 per cent).

As far as the role of the spousal relationship is concerned, it has to be underlined that in Italy most older people still attribute a fundamental importance to their marriage, a situation confirmed by the relatively low number of single, divorced or separated among the over 65 year olds (Eurostat 2000). Among the changes occurring after retirement, the opportunity to spend more time with one's spouse is considered as extremely 'relevant' by one older person out of five, and the spouse's death is among the most frequently quoted events that symbolically indicate 'the entry into old age' (Palomba *et al.* 2001).

The other pivot of Italian family life is children and 89 per cent of older people have at least one child, 41 per cent two, in most cases living near their parents' house (17 per cent in the same building, 21 per cent in the same neighbourhood, 41 per cent in the same town). When children move from their parents' house this does not interrupt family relations, not even in terms of daily habits (33 per cent of older people usually have their lunch and supper with their children, 53 per cent do it sometimes; 73 per cent always spend Christmas with their children, 26 per cent always spend their summer holidays with them). Data from ISTAT (2001c) similarly show that contacts with parents are still very frequent even when the children make up a new family unit (54 per cent of the over-65s meet their children every day, and 38 per cent telephone them every day). By contrast, only 17 per cent of fathers and 20 per cent of mothers lose contact with their children and never get in touch with them.

The great majority of older people (71 per cent) have grandchildren (ISTAT 2001c) and this relationship is of great importance in the life of the over

65 year olds: 36 per cent of them look after them 'regularly' and 42 per cent 'sometimes' (Palomba *et al.* 2001). The help and protection they give to their grandchildren allows older people to regain an important and active role, and to play a useful and, at times, indispensable part in family life again. This seems to be confirmed by the fact that older people who live in a large family, including those where grandchildren are present, enjoy, on average, better living conditions, both from the economic and the emotional point of view (SPI-CGIL 1997).

The comparative findings emerging from the ESAW study (Burholt *et al.* 2003: 24ff) confirm the central role played by multigenerational living arrangements for older Italians. They live much more often with children, parents and siblings – but not with grandchildren – and they are much more seldom alone than older people in Central and Northern European countries. The high frequency of this 'extended family based' household pattern seems to be justified by the relatively high satisfaction expressed by older Italians, together with Dutch and British respondents, with regard to their family relationships. A direct consequence of this situation is the relatively high number of opportunities to talk and have contact and conversations with other people reported by older Italians, both with cohabiting and non-cohabiting persons (probably relatives belonging to the family's extended network). Thus it is surprising that a relatively high percentage (13 per cent) of older Italians report both 'not having anyone they could trust and confide in' and 'feeling lonely'. This negative assessment is confirmed by the relatively low levels of satisfaction characterizing older Italians with regard to overall family and friendship relationships, but is contradicted by the higher proportion of Italians answering that, if necessary, they could count on someone who would take care of them as long as needed. This apparent contradiction might be explained by a culturally specific content attributed by older Italians to concepts such as 'trust', 'confidence' and 'loneliness', which in their minds could be separated by 'availability of help'. Also the feelings of (lack of) trust and of loneliness could well reflect the condition of those Italians who do not feel 'normal' compared to the local standards of accentuated familism found in the country.

Friends, neighbourhood and other support networks

Less importance is attributed to friends, neighbours and other support networks, compared with the family. The most recent available data show that the number of older people who meet their friends daily does not significantly decrease, but, on the contrary, for women, increases even beyond the age of 75 (Table 8.3). However, there is also an increase in the number of people, mostly women, who, with growing age, cannot meet their friends any longer or who declare they have no friends at all.

Table 8.3 Over 65 year old population by frequency of meeting with friends and gender (%)

	Males			Females		
	60–4	65–74	Over 75	60–4	65–74	Over 75
Every day	25.5	28.1	21.3	2.8	12.3	13.4
Every once in a while	68.8	63.5	60.9	84.8	72.5	60.1
Never	4.2	5.8	11.7	7.9	9.5	16.4
Has no friends	1.5	2.6	6.1	4.5	5.7	9.2

Source: ISTAT (2001d).

The ESAW data confirm this picture. Older Italians, together with Austrians and UK respondents, complain more often than other older Europeans of not 'being able to see friends and relatives as often as they want' (Burholt 2003: 25ff), a result that might also partly explain why they do not seem particularly satisfied with their friendship relationships. On the other hand, it has to be underlined that older Italians, while reporting being less satisfied about their contacts and relationships (see also previous paragraph), do actually have much more frequent contacts with friends and neighbours than other Europeans. This might therefore reveal a basic Italian tendency to both feel and express dissatisfaction rather than any real differences.

Participation and social integration

Volunteering, religious attendance and political participation

With advancing age a reduction in the rate of participation of older Italians in organized activities and volunteering and also in some social and cultural associations takes place (Table 8.4, col. 1–3). This confirms a previously observed trend that this is particularly true for men (Sgritta and Saporiti 1997, 1998: 29). When leaving employment, participation in community life tends to decrease. Despite a low participation rate in trade unions and professional organizations, older people (Table 8.4, col. 4) continue to feel represented much more than the rest of the population (CNEL 2000).

Table 8.4 Over 55 year olds participating in social activities and frequency of religious practice, 2000 (per 100 persons of same age)

Age group	1 Meetings in ecological associations or pacifist and social rights movements (a).		2 Meetings in cultural, recreational or similar associations (a).		3 Free activity for volunteer or similar associations (a).		4 Free activity for a trade union (a).		5 Frequency of religious practice: never		6 at least once a week (b)	
	M	F	M	F	M	F	M	F	M	F	M	F
55–9	2.1	1.2	11.8	7.6	16.2	12.4	3.8	1.0	15.9	7.3	29.1	49.6
60–4	1.6	0.7	9.5	6.1	13.4	10.9	2.5	0.6	13.4	7.0	31.5	57.8
65–74	1.0	0.3	7.7	4.4	8.7	6.4	1.1	0.4	16.5	8.0	35.2	62.2
75 and over	0.6	0.1	4.7	2.0	3.3	2.8	0.9	0.0	22.3	18.1	36.2	49.9

Notes:

(a) at least once a year

(b) the original answers were: 'every day', 'more than once a week', 'once a week', 'more than once a month', 'sometimes in a year' and 'never'; this modality sums the frequencies of the first three answers.

Source: ISTAT (2001d).

As far as religious practices are concerned (Table 8.4, col. 5–6), the data refer to 'going to church' (and not praying or carrying out other religious activities). There is an increase in the number who never go to church, especially among people over 75, an age at which there is a remarkable reduction in female participation, while regular male participation increases even in the oldest age group.

In older age a decline also takes place in political participation, even in relatively passive activities, although participation remains higher for men in all age groups (Table 8.5). Seventy per cent of women over 75 never talk about politics and 55 per cent never show any interest in it (Table 8.6), compared with 39 per cent and 26 per cent respectively for men, confirming both gender differences and the strong age-related reduction in interest in politics.

The involvement of older Italians in volunteering activities is much lower than that of older people from Northern European countries (Drooglever Fortuijin *et al.* 2003: 15–21). However, when they are involved, they provide their volunteer support, usually of one kind only, on a much more frequent basis (72 per cent at least weekly), thus revealing Italy's characteristic tendency to be what Dekker and Van den Broek (1998) have called a 'parochial kind of civil society'. Most Italian volunteers belong to the middle and upper socio-economic classes in terms of income and educational level and are concentrated in the younger age cohorts. On the whole, though, the level of older Italians' overall wellbeing does not seem to be very highly correlated with their involvement in volunteer activities.

Participation in organizations and clubs: the third age universities

One of the most important cultural developments involving older people in Italy in the last few years is the institution of the universities of the third age. The first ones started mainly during the 1980s but became more widespread mostly during the 1990s, especially in the Centre and in the North of Italy. They seem to meet a double need: on one hand, they provide the opportunity to learn subjects and skills, thus contributing to preventing the risk of social exclusion (Frey 2001a: 2); on the other hand, they foster a form of active involvement that helps in facing the emotional and social difficulties following retirement (Foschi and Barbini 2000).

It is indeed true that the risk of exclusion due to the lack of education is particularly high among Italian older people, owing to their low average level of education, since only 3 per cent of over 65 year olds have a university degree and only 6.5 per cent a high school diploma (ISTAT 2001e). These percentages

Table 8.5 Over 55 year olds participating in political activities 2000 (per 100 persons of same age and sex)

Age group	1 Participation in a political meeting.		2 Participation in a political demonstration.		3 Listening at political debate.		4 Free activity for a political party.		5 Has donated money to a political party.	
	M	F	M	F	M	F	M	F	M	F
55–9	9.7	2.9	3.8	2.1	33.4	18.9	3.4	0.9	5.4	2.2
60–4	7.1	1.6	3.5	1.4	28.5	13.4	2.4	0.7	4.0	1.2
65–74	6.6	0.9	2.4	1.0	23.1	10.3	1.7	0.5	3.3	1.0
75 and over	3.8	0.6	2.0	0.3	16.0	6.7	0.8	–	2.3	0.4

Source: ISTAT (2001d).

Table 8.6 Frequency with which over 55 year olds talk and get information about politics, 2000 (per 100 persons of same age and sex)

Age group	Talks politics:						Gets information on politics:					
	Every day		Sometimes in a month		Never		Every day		Sometimes in a month		Never	
	M	F	M	F	M	F	M	F	M	F	M	F
55–59	14.6	6.6	16.4	14.2	17.0	44.0	51.7	29.0	5.4	8.5	10.2	30.5
60–4	12.5	4.6	18.2	12.0	19.7	54.9	49.4	26.9	7.3	7.4	11.8	38.2
65–74	10.2	3.2	16.7	9.1	27.6	60.6	42.3	23.7	7.2	6.8	17.2	43.7
75 and over	6.5	1.6	12.7	7.5	39.3	70.5	38.1	16.3	7.0	5.2	25.7	55.1

Source: ISTAT (2001d).

are bound to rise in the next few years, and among people between 55 and 64 years of age are likely to reach 5 per cent and 17 per cent respectively, although they still remain very low compared to the average rate of the OECD countries. Despite several initiatives that have been undertaken to foster the education of older people in Italy (Frey 1997), most efforts have proven to be inadequate. The teaching methods and the content of courses are particularly inappropriate and inadequate and are unable to promote knowledge and learning skills in older people (Frey 2001a: 10).

In this context, the universities of the third age are one of the biggest and most important initiatives in Italy for the education and updating of those who did not have any opportunity to attend a higher school when they were young. The activities run by these institutions, while actively contributing to delaying the ageing process in the participants, also promote the development of more active forms of social life in old age by fostering participation in associations with the pleasure of sharing experiences, thus promoting a more positive and active image of older age (Frey 1997: 54).

While in the past the degree of education among the university of the third age students was higher than average (Turrini 1987; Frey 1997: 5), recent studies show a trend towards an increase in the participation of older people with lower educational levels (Grammarota 1996). Among the reasons why older people enrol in these initiatives, the most important are the wish to overcome some of the limits implied in old age, the desire to increase personal psychophysical autonomy, the search for new opportunities of socialization and enjoyment as well as the wish for a higher level of culture and scientific knowledge (Frey 1997: 60). Despite some negative aspects, such as difficulties inherent in the volunteer activity and, above all, the lack of teaching strategies suitable to meet to older students' expectations, the contribution of this experience to the quality of life of many older Italians, on the whole, is positive.

Isolation and loneliness

The fact that about a quarter of all older people live alone as a consequence of new, more individualized forms of living arrangements does not necessarily mean a correspondingly widespread increase in loneliness among older people, as partly confirmed by the abovementioned studies on 'intimacy at a distance'. Nevertheless, some population groups are at risk of loneliness, in particular widows, especially in the northern part of the country, where the role of the extended family is less strong, thus contributing to the feeling of loneliness in the case of loss of a spouse (EURISPES-SIP 1993). Isolation and poor social relations have often been found to be associated, especially in older people with low levels of autonomy and with a higher risk of poverty (Delai 1998: 61). The risk of loneliness might also derive from the *frustration* that sometimes characterizes the post-retirement phase, even when psychophysical conditions remain good, due to a feeling of marginalization from social and productive life (IRP-CNR 2001), which many older persons, especially men, try to face through an approach that is still based on criteria and methods typical of the working world, instead of looking for new forms of social participation (Urbani 1991: 218).

There is a series of initiatives intended to tackle the problem of loneliness, fostering social integration and overcoming the isolating effects that the transformation of family structures and retirement might have on older people. Among these initiatives – which include the third age universities – there is the wide range of social, cultural and recreational centres for older people, which facilitate regular contact among older people living in the same neighbourhood. Another common way to fight loneliness and isolation is in confessional groups, which represent for many older people not only a support in the most intimate and traditional religious practices (like praying or going to Church), but also a very important source of social contact within community life.

A similar role is played by volunteer work but this is a task accessible only to older people in fairly good health, for whom it can constitute a good preventive measure to escape loneliness (Livraghi 1997). 'Banks of time' are an innovative form of volunteer work (Olini 1999), as they are based on the free exchange of work and services among people of all ages, thus actively contributing to interpersonal and intergenerational socialization, especially in the northern regions of the country, where they are more common (Presidenza del Consiglio dei Ministri, 2000: 145).

The role of services in quality of life

Health services

Older people represent the main users of health services. Older Italians might resort to health services more often than older citizens of other countries due to a 'fiscal exemption effect', that is the fact that over 65-year-olds with a family income lower than 36,000 euros are by law exempted from payment of health-care services (Legge no. 537/1993). Although some studies ascribe only a marginal role to this phenomenon (SPI-CGIL/CER 1997: 39), there is a larger use of services and of pharmaceutical drugs in older age groups (Table 8.7, col. 1–2).

Table 8.7 Over 55 year olds' use of medicines and GPs, 2000
(per 100 persons of same age and sex)

Age group	Has used medicines in the last two days		Has resorted to the GP for health problems	
	M	F	M	F
55–9	38.7	48.1	79.2	82.4
60–4	47.8	55.9	79.6	85.8
65–74	61.2	67.6	85.9	88.7
75 and over	76.2	77.5	90.0	90.6

Source: ISTAT (2001b).

Within the Italian healthcare system a central role is played by the GP (Table 8.7, cols 3–6). This is the profession responsible for supplying free medical care to patients in all age groups (up to a maximum of 1500 per GP), with whom most older patients have built up a relationship throughout their life, referring to him or her as the 'family doctor'. People normally ask for the GP's help in case of need or for routine check ups, and when necessary for bureaucratic reasons (such as prescriptions or the issue of certificates). Thus the relationship with their GP is a substantial element of the QoL of older Italians in the health field (SPI-CGIL-CER 1997).

The hospital is another important institution in the healthcare of older people (Table 8.8, cols 1–2). The increasing admissions trend is inverted for men over 80, when longer hospital stays are recorded (col. 3). As some associations in defence of patients' rights have already pointed out in the past (Santanera *et al.* 1994), this seems to show a lower willingness on the part of hospital administration to admit older patients because they require longer stays (Cariani *et al.* 1997: 114), which mean higher costs for the hospitals, whose services since the early 1990s have been subject to reimbursement according to the Diagnosis Related Group (DRG) system (Decreto Ministero Sanità 1994). This is confirmed by the fact that the use of emergency care units and of the first aid stations does not decrease for men over 80 (ISTAT 2001b).

As far as the accessibility of care services is concerned many older people do not seem to be adequately informed about the existence and the possibility of using some services, in particular those of home care and day hospital, especially in the south of the country (SPI-CGIL/CER 1997: 40). Older people also generally favour public health services rather than privately owned

Table 8.8 Number of hospital admissions and average length of hospital stay among over 55 year olds, 2000 (%)

Age group	1 Number of admissions (a).		2 Persons with at least one admission (a).		3 Average number of days in hospital (b).	
	M	F	M	F	M	F
55–64	5.3	5.7	4.6	4.0	8.9	7.8
65–9	9.6	6.5	6.5	5.4	7.3	9.5
70–4	9.3	7.8	7.9	6.4	10.1	10.8
75–9	15.2	8.5	12.3	7.3	10.3	9.0
80 and over	13.6	9.8	11.7	8.5	13.5	10.5

Notes:
(a) for 100 persons
(b) average length of stay
Source: ISTAT (2001b).

ones (CNEL 2000). This is particularly evident in the case of laboratory tests, while it is less so for specialist treatments (SPI-CGIL/CER 1997), and is probably due mainly to economic factors, while the length of waiting lists becomes important when older people resort to private paid healthcare services (CENSIS/Forum per la ricerca biomedica 2002, Table 37). Waiting lists represent a crucial area where measures should be implemented in order to improve QoL in older age as far as health services are concerned.

ESAW data show that, on average, older Italians see a doctor (or other health professional) much more often than other Europeans (except for Austrians), and they also make relatively frequent use of inpatient hospital services, while they resort less frequently to nursing homes and rehabilitation centres (Ferring *et al.* 2003: 20–2, 34–6). They also differ from other older Europeans with regard to the use of aids and prosthetics, reporting much less frequent use of glasses (84 per cent against an overall average of 92 per cent) and hearing aids (2 per cent against 6–7 per cent), but also of other devices such as partial or complete dentures, canes, walking frames, wheelchairs and other physical aids, showing (together with Sweden) a relatively high percentage of people using no aids at all (57 per cent, against an overall average of 51 per cent). In terms of QoL, this low use of health services and aids is felt by many older Italians as a lack of appropriate care, because almost one-fifth of them (that is double the overall average) 'feel the need for additional medical care and treatment in correspondence to a lower vision and hearing quality and an overall worse health status' (see Chapter 3). On the other hand, Italians seem to feel less need for further 'supportive or prosthetic devices', which might, however, reveal a lack of knowledge of the improvement such devices might mean for their everyday life, and report lower rates (compared for instance to the UK and Sweden) of people feeling unable to pay for their healthcare expenses (Lamura *et al.* 2003: 28–9).

Social services

Despite the fact that people over 65 comprise 52 per cent of the recipients of social services (Ancitel 2001), the spread of such services specifically aimed at this age group in Italy is rather low. This is evident both for the home care services and for older people's residential homes, which are used by a smaller proportion of older people (1 per cent and 2 per cent respectively) than in Northern and Central Europe (OCSE 1996; Gori 2001a: 28). Where these and other social care services exist, another Italian anomaly is the high amount of the users' contributions to the cost of these services, which in Italy amounts on average to 50 per cent, a much higher proportion than in other European countries (Frey 2001b).

Furthermore, particularly with regard to the provision of home care services, great inequalities can be observed among the various regions, in terms both of implementation of the services and of integration among the different home care services, to the disadvantage of the rural and southern areas, where social services are often offered in the form of more or less regular sums of money (Ancitel 2001). This helps to explain why the users of social services are mostly concentrated in the south of the country, mainly as recipients of monetary transfers.

Thus there is a strong latent demand for social services in kind, which is shown by the fact that, among the services most requested by older people, a primary role is played by home care services (15.2 per cent), admission to nursing homes (14.6 per cent), summer holidays (12.8 per cent), telemedical aids (9.9 per cent) or meals on wheels (9.5 per cent), while economic allowances or benefits such as, for instance, reduced transport fares (8.1 per cent), represent only a second choice (Ancitel 2001). This reflects the existence among older Italians of a strong demand for support and counselling in deciding how to choose the most suitable services for the care needs arising in older age to avoid being left alone in the market for private services, which in Italy is relatively little developed and characterized by high levels of undeclared work, mainly in the form of foreign immigrants providing home care.

This demand for support has been met partly due to the tendency (which is consolidating in Italy and in other Southern European countries) to consider social services for older people no longer as a form of intervention only for the poor or as only consisting of financial aid (as these allowances have existed at a national level as disability or care allowances since 1980) (Lamura *et al.* 2001). As a matter of fact, the introduction of alternative forms of assistance such as vouchers on the part of public administrations (municipal administrations, regions or ASL) is becoming increasingly common (Ancitel 2001). In the 1990s this kind of intervention was widely implemented in the north and in the central regions of Italy (where about 40 per cent of municipalities and ASL use them, compared with 12 per cent of municipal administrations and no ASL in the south), thus giving rise again to a very uneven distribution of such forms of support (Gori 2001b: 80; Gori and Torri 2001).

Social security

Although the Italian social security system is comparable, in terms of degree of protection of social risks, to those in force in most industrialized countries, the presence of some insufficiently protected risks and some overprotected ones (OECD 2000a) illustrates the necessity of major modifications to guarantee greater equity in the allocation of resources among the older population. Several proposals have been considered including tax reductions and the introduction of a means-tested, universal guaranteed minimum income or of a universal but non-means tested citizen's income, for every citizen (De Vincenti and Minelli 2001: 86). Another option, which has been realized through the Financial Law 2002 (law no. 448/2001, art. 38) is an increase in the amount of the lowest pensions from the previous minimum of 393 euros to the current level of 516 euros per month. This increase has been in force since the beginning of 2002 for about 600,000 retired people, and for a further several hundred thousand recipients since the end of the same year, according to the entitlements which are (a) being older than 70 (a limit which can be reduced to 60 in case of total disability, or to 65 if social contributions have been paid up) and (b) earning a yearly income lower than 6714 euros (or 11,271 euros in the case of married couples) (Pierpaoli 2002).

Life satisfaction and subjective wellbeing

Family relationships (Table 8.9) are the aspect of life that is considered to be the most satisfactory among older people, without any remarkable difference

Table 8.9 Proportion of over 55 year olds 'very satisfied' or 'satisfied' with main aspects of life, 2000 (per 100 persons of same age and sex)

Age group	Economic conditions		Health		Family relationships		Friendships		Leisure time		Work	
	M	F	M	F	M	F	M	F	M	F	M	F
55–9	61.3	59.1	77.6	74.4	89.7	92.2	84.4	78.7	64.1	59.5	76.1	78.1
60–4	59.1	55.7	75.2	65.7	91.3	90.1	84.4	77.9	70.2	66.0	71.1	78.6
65–74	61.0	55.8	64.3	57.0	90.4	88.8	82.4	74.7	76.5	67.9	80.3	78.8
75 and over	59.4	54.0	49.7	45.2	87.9	87.2	73.0	64.7	72.7	64.2	81.6	68.8

Source: ISTAT (2001d).

in terms of gender or age. On the contrary, health and economic conditions seem to be the source of the highest dissatisfaction – health in particular – for men over 65 and women over 60, and finance throughout all age groups. Confirming a trend already observed for self-perceived health (Chapter 3), women appear to be relatively less satisfied than men in all aspects of life, and in particular when dealing with friendships, free time and work (Presidenza del Consiglio dei Ministri 2000: 70). In the last case, however, dissatisfaction is limited only to the over-75s, while in the age group between 55 and 65 an opposite trend is recorded, probably linked to the loss of an active social role on the part of men on the verge of retirement.

These data support the traditional model of Italian men, which is more projected towards relationships outside the family, while women are more concentrated on the home and family relationships. Men's satisfaction with family relationships is higher if their wife is still alive and if their children have already left the parents' household (married men with no children scored the highest levels of satisfaction in all age groups, while lowest male satisfaction scores were recorded in the case of those with children still living with them and of spouse's death, both especially among the over-70s) (Aureli and Baldazzi 1999).

For women, on the other hand, especially in the oldest age groups, the condition of being the only parent is correlated with the highest satisfaction with family life. This confirms the assumption that, while the central family relationship for Italian women is based on their children, especially if they cohabit with them, older men consider this cohabitation as a signal of their reduced independence, and hence a source of worry, even if not to the extent reached in the case of the loss of their wife, the pivot of their family and relational life, which causes the most substantial reduction in men's QoL.

Earlier research showed that 80 per cent of older people were 'absolutely satisfied' or 'quite satisfied' with their present life, while the percentage of those who were 'utterly dissatisfied' was lower than 3 per cent of the total sample (EURISPES 1993). The study pointed out, moreover, the central role played by several factors in influencing the level of life satisfaction in old age: the level of education (the higher the education level, the higher the satisfaction) and work (older people who never worked are the most dissatisfied). Despite the importance of variables such as gender, marital status, family size and composition, finance and housing, health was confirmed, once again, as the one that mostly influences older people's QoL: 33

per cent of them consider good health as the main reason for their satisfaction with life whereas 23 per cent attribute it to being self-sufficient. Within this study, a central role was also associated with 'affections and personal relations', which rated second among the factors codetermining their satisfaction level.

The centrality of health and health-related issues in general for older people's QoL is confirmed by other recent surveys, whose results, however, are not comparable due to the use of quite different research methodologies. A study of the Italian National Council for Economy and Work (CNEL), for example, has pointed out that the level of attention older people devote to the problem of health is equalled only by that devoted to the 'pension issue' (CNEL 2000: 4); while according to the survey conducted by SPI/CGIL (1997: 50) housing represents, after health, the second major problem (but it is rated first, even before health, by 16 per cent of the older population). In the same study the issue of leisure time was rated third after health and housing, and the problem of personal security followed in fourth place. In answer to the question 'what are the main concerns for an old person?' 38 per cent said 'the loss of physical autonomy' and 25 per cent 'the loss of a beloved person', compared with which concerns about finance, loneliness and retirement received almost negligible ratings, especially in the over 75 year old age group.

The ESAW findings show that, for Europe as a whole, material security and health status are the most important predictors of life satisfaction and, together with social support resources, also of self-worth (Ferring *et al.* 2003a). Cross-national differences are pronounced, and for older Italians, the most important factors for QoL are the social support resources, followed by health and material security on the same level, life activities being the least relevant (but still significant). Compared with the overall European situation, life satisfaction of older Italians is more strongly associated with the functioning of their support networks and less to economic wellbeing. It is moderately related to health status, and slightly more strongly related to life activities. A final relevant finding of the ESAW study is that both age and gender have an indirect influence on life satisfaction and self-worth, which for older Italians is explained through lower material security, worse health and less social support in older age groups, a similar pattern also being followed for women, with the exception of life activities: Italian older women are more active.

Inequalities and variations in quality of life

In almost all areas analysed in this chapter and Chapter 3, differences in terms of QoL can be observed, mainly with regard to geographical area and gender but also in terms of age, income and occupational group. Information regarding racial or ethnic differentiation in old age is almost absent, partly due to the very low number of foreign immigrants and ethnic minorities in the older age groups.

Territorial inequalities

Older people living in the northern regions of the country, as with the whole population of those regions, generally enjoy better economic conditions and higher income levels (SPI-CGIL/CER 1997), can count on a better organized network of health and social care services (Gori 2001a; 2001b), including nursing homes and other residential structures, and have a higher involvement in volunteer work and other organized forms of social life (Sgritta and Saporiti 1998: 37) than those in the south. A more in-depth look at this general picture shows that in northern Italy the older population have lower incomes than the younger age groups. Whereas in the south the very high youth unemployment rates, together with the higher importance attached to the redistributive role of the family, allow older people to play meaningful roles, both economically and socially, within local society and family structures (SPI-CGIL/CER 1997).

Recent data show that, while urban areas, especially in the north of the country, provide a growing range of home care services and a good range of other public and private services, the demographic contraction of some rural areas, especially those located on the Appenines (the mountain chain that crosses the whole country from north to south), is leading to the creation of 'elderly only villages', doomed to extinction in a few decades, and currently characterized by an increasingly poor range of social and economic services, which dramatically threatens the QoL of all the older residents (Golini and Bruno 1999).

Gender inequalities

We have already emphasized that women's family experience is mainly one of loneliness, due to high incidence of widowhood, a condition that contributes to a stronger perception of low security and leads many women to take precautions more often than men, both outdoors and at home. Gender differences seem to affect all aspects of life; older women use new technology less frequently, prefer to cycle or walk rather than drive a car, and use fewer services like banks, the post office or the hospital, but are much bigger users of other healthcare services (like the GP) and of medicines.

A major source of gender differentiation is employment because of the economic consequences that low participation in the labour market have in older age. Due to the large proportion of housewives and of early retired women (8.4 per cent of total versus 0.4 per cent for men), more than one-third of women (36.5 per cent) cannot count on personal resources to live on, compared with 0.1 per cent of men (Livraghi 1996: 87).

Future research priorities

In the light of the above evidence the following suggestions can be formulated for future research in Italy. Future housing studies should try to focus not only on the objective characteristics of buildings – on which data are relatively abundant – but also on the subjective aspects, or how to include the perception of the older person in this evaluation, because for many older people an old-fashioned and structurally poor dwelling might appear to be far preferable to recently built and technologically advanced accommodation. A further, related issue needing more in-depth investigation is the analysis of the circumstances of the most frequent domestic accidents of which older people are victims. Security is also an issue of paramount importance that deserves to be studied more thoroughly, in particular with regard to the needs of older women who often live alone and feel threatened both within and outside the domestic environment.

Another aspect that deserves attention is the attitudes of older people and potential family caregivers towards the use of nursing homes and other residential facilities, in the light of the growing difficulty that Italian families experience in ensuring adequate care at home. It is crucial to analyse how to improve the integration of these facilities in the local community by opening internal services to the general public and facilitating residents' use of community services.

It is necessary for future research to develop a greater connection between studies based on the subjective perceptions of older people and objective, clinical evaluations provided by professionals, in order to understand better the implications of health deficits for the accomplishment of everyday life activities. There is also a need to reach greater comparability of results at an international level through the use of similar, standardized assessment tools and statistical instruments.

The transformation of family structure has been widely studied from a demographic point of view but sociological and qualitative information on older people's families remains scarce. In particular, it would be interesting to study older people who live alone in order to better understand what QoL means for this growing group of older Italians. In Italy literature about neighbourhood and friends in old age is not very abundant and thus deserves greater importance in the future.

Last but not least, a need that emerges from the whole analysis carried out for this book regards the necessity of being able to count on reliable data and in-depth analyses distinguished by gender as well as socio-economic and occupational history, but also ethnicity, in the light of the growing number of foreign immigrants reaching old age in Italy in recent years. The identification of more precise outcomes in terms of QoL in older age – taking the example of what has already been made available mainly in the field of healthcare, but within a broader and less health-centred conceptual framework – would benefit greatly from such data, making the improvement of older Italians' wellbeing a less abstract goal.

Conclusion

This chapter shows that, despite the deep demographic and sociocultural changes experienced by the Italian family in the last few decades, this institution still represents the main source of social support for most older Italians, who live much more often than other Europeans in multigenerational households and maintain daily contacts with children and other close relatives. It is no surprise, therefore, that the role played by other social networks – such as those based on friendship, neighbourhood or volunteer and community based involvement – seems to be less pronounced, at least in terms of subjective satisfaction. Although some recent mass phenomena, such as the 'third age universities' and the retirees trade unions, show the need of many older Italians to have a less familistic approach to life. As far as services are concerned, it has to be emphasized that the general expectation of most Italians in older age is to have to find personal solutions to solve their health-related and/or social problems, as the widespread phenomenon of hiring personal assistants to care for frail older people clearly shows.

However, some signs of change are evident and future research will have to try to understand them, especially in the fields of accessibility of services, housing, the transition to retirement and the strengthening of non-kin social networks.

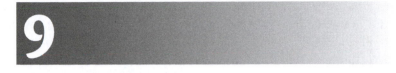

9

The Netherlands: quality of life in old age II

Annemarie Peeters, Beitske Bouwman and
Kees Knipscheer

Family and support networks

Personal relationships are important to older people and have a significant impact upon their wellbeing (House and Kahn 1985; Knipscheer *et al.* 1995). During the lifecourse there are constant changes in relationship patterns and one of the most remarkable of these is the consistent rise in one-person households. Forecasts for the Netherlands indicate that this trend will continue in the future (De Beer, De Jong and Visser 1993; Knipscheer *et al.* 1995). Given that wives tend to outlive their husbands, the majority of older people living in one-person households are widows. The increasing number of older people who are living on their own implies an increasing number of older people in vulnerable positions (Knipscheer *et al.* 1995).

According to the NESTOR and LASA surveys[1] (1995) more than 80 per cent of men aged under 75 live with a partner. Among the youngest old, many of these couples have children in the household as well, but this category decreases rapidly in size among older age groups. After age 75 the proportion of men living with a partner decreases, but of the men aged 85 to 89 almost half live with a partner. The proportion of older men living alone is stable at around 10 per cent until age 80, but increases to about 30 per cent among the oldest age group (Liefbroer and de Jong Gierveld 1995).

For a number of years, research has shown that a confidant, such as a partner or a friend, is an important source of support. NESTOR figures show that respondents living with a partner have more relationships and more support exchanges than those who live alone. This does not mean that living alone in itself has negative implications for the network. For example, older people who live alone have relatively more neighbours and friends in their close support network in comparison with others (Knipscheer *et al.* 1995: 181). It looks like age plays an important role in giving and receiving support. The older one is, the fewer relationships one has and the more limited the intensity of exchanges within the network. Older respondents receive more instrumental support and less emotional support from fewer network members than younger respondents. However, caution is necessary when interpreting the age differences as change because these results are based on cross-sectional data.

It is well established that QoL in old age strongly depends on intergenerational family solidarity (Antonucci *et al.* 1996; Bengtson *et al.* 1996; Tesch-Romer *et al.* 2001). Many studies have focused on the relationship between older people and their children. It is known that children are important: older people are exchanging a lot of support with them (Antonucci *et al.* 1996; Bengtson *et al.* 1996; Tesch-Romer *et al.* 1996). Data show that older parents are not isolated from their siblings and their children. On average about 75 per cent of older people have monthly contact with at least one of their siblings and about 15 per cent have interactions with four of them. Two-thirds of older people have at least one of their siblings living within a travelling distance of less than 30 minutes. As expected, interaction with children is more frequent and a higher proportion of children live nearby than siblings. More than 90 per cent of parents have weekly contact with at least one child, and over 50 per cent have three or more children with whom they interact monthly or more often. More than 85 per cent of the parents have at least one child living within a travelling distance of less than 30 minutes (Knipscheer *et al.* 1995: 177). The suggestion that older people who live alone are lonely and isolated does not do justice to the fact that most have relationships with other people.

Forty per cent of 55 to 59 year olds have at least one parent, over 90 per cent have at least one brother or sister and roughly the same percentage have one or more children. More than half have grandchildren. Up to the age of 75 there is little change in the number of older people who have children and/or brothers and sisters. By this age, the proportion with grandchildren has risen to 80 per cent. A majority of older people in the Netherlands (73 per cent) are part of a family of three or more generations; 12 per cent have neither parents nor children (Dykstra and Knipscheer 1995: 53). The proportion of older people who have four or more brothers or sisters (this figure has been chosen because this applies to around half of those aged 55 to 59) declines as these relatives die. After the age of 75, the ranks have thinned so

Table 9.1 Older people and their relatives 1992 (%)

	55–9 yrs	60–4 yrs	65–9 yrs	70–4 yrs	75–9 yrs	80–4 yrs	85–9 yrs
Parent(s)	38	20	9	4	2	1	
Brothers and sisters	93	90	92	89	85	75	62
Child(ren)	88	87	87	85	86	79	73
Grandchild(ren)	48	65	75	79	83	76	75
Four or more brothers and sisters	47	42	40	32	24	20	10
Three or more children	44	49	51	48	51	45	43

Source: SCP 1996; Nestor-LSN'92: calculation by Dykstra and Knipscheer (1995).

much that the number of older people without brothers and sisters (-in-law) increases to 40 per cent. The proportion of older people with children is also lower above the age of 75. This is because of the relatively large number of women in this age group who have never married or had children, and because of parents outliving their children (Dykstra and Call 1997). The Nestor study also counted people as part of the network if the respondents indicated that they were important to them and they had regular contact with them. Children and other relatives each appear to account for around a quarter of the network. After this, neighbours and friends were mentioned most often (12 per cent and 10 per cent). Fellow members of organizations (including the Church), current and ex-colleagues and acquaintances were also found to be significant, each accounting for around 5 per cent of the network (Van Tilburg 1995: 87). Over three-quarters of the children of the respondents and some 40 per cent of their brothers and sisters (-in-law) were regarded by the respondents as part of their network (Dykstra 1995: 109). The network of those aged 55 to 59 with children was found to consist of 14 people on average, whereas that of their contemporaries without children was some-what smaller, at nine. The network appeared to be smaller and less diverse the older the age group in question. Given the categories in the network that show the sharpest decline (brothers, sisters and friends), the main cause of this is the death of the individual's contemporaries.

Those without children have more friends, neighbours and other relatives in their network than those with children. Neighbours and other relatives are important to people in the oldest age groups, as they consistently comprise half of the individuals in the network. The networks of older people in residential homes are clearly smaller than those of people who live independently. This applies to all the categories of the network identified. As with people living independently, those without children have more friends, neighbours and other relatives in their network.

Neighbourhood support and friendships

Networks also include neighbours and friends who, with slightly more distant relatives, are more likely to form part of the network of those who live alone, while children (-in-law) and brothers and sisters (-in-law) are less likely to figure. In comparison with friends, neighbours give less emotional support and a lot of instrumental support. Friends offer more emotional than instrumental support.

Older people living alone in urbanized areas turn out to have considerably less contact with their neighbours than their peers in rural areas. This minor contact is entirely or partly compensated for by contacts at a greater distance. Less neighbourhood contact does have consequences for the possibilities of support in daily activities in and around the household (Fokkema and de Jong Gierveld 1999). Older people in rural areas are strongly neighbourhood oriented, while older people in urbanized areas are more focused on the world outside their direct environment. Their networks are less locally oriented. However, this means that in proportion to their network size they receive little instrumental support – for this type of support closeness is an important condition (Fokkema and de Jong Gierveld 1999). Different studies show that friendship is more important for older women than for older men. Women tend to have more contacts with friends in advanced years and they often use support from friends for coping with the loss of their partner (Stevens 1998).

Grandparenting

The change in timing of life events like earlier marriage and earlier and more closely spaced children have made grandparenthood a more youthful role and have given it a new cultural image. There is a lot of diversity of grandparenting styles. According to NESTOR data (1995) 68.8 per cent of the respondents (N = 4137) have at least one grandchild, and 10.4 per cent have at least one great grandchild (Dykstra and Knipscheer 1995).

Spruytte et al. (1998) looked at the relationship between the conceptions of being a grandparent and the psychological wellbeing of the older people. The research was conducted with 250 Dutch-speaking Belgians. The grandparents were in general very positive about the relationship with their oldest grandchild. Items like feeling happy about the relationship with their grandchild, feeling responsible for helping the grandchild and feeling a worthy grandparent were endorsed by almost all grandparents. All grandparents generally reported wellbeing for all dimensions.

Participation and social integration

Participation is a very broad concept. Terms such as 'voluntary work', 'community participation' and 'social participation' are difficult to distinguish from each other in the various studies. Lameiro Garcia and Van Rijsselt (1992: 84 in SCP 1998) therefore conclude, in their study of social participation, that this is a 'container concept'. Knipscheer et al. (1995: 24 in SCP 1998) define participation broadly as 'everything which is not paid employment or personal care' (the definition is used this chapter).

Political participation

Older people vote more frequently than people aged under 55. In 1994, for example (according to a survey that generally overestimates the number of voters), around 90 per cent of older people (over-55s) voted during the parliamentary elections compared with 80 per cent of those aged 35 to 54. These differences between age categories remain after correction for differences in education level or labour market position. Although older people vote more frequently than under-55s, they protest less often and have less often filled in a petition or taken part in a demonstration. However, this appears to be more of a generation effect than an age effect; future older people will have taken part in significantly more protests than present-day older people. Older people have contacted a politician or tried to call on the help of an official body just as frequently as younger people. According to the Time Use Survey (TBO),[2] 7 per cent of the population aged 35 and over play an active part in political activities. Older people (over-55s) are less frequently involved in such activities than younger people (SCP 1998: 149–50).

Social participation

The membership rate of associations or community organizations decreases with increasing age: 74 per cent of those aged under 75 are members, compared with 50 per cent of over-75s. The biggest difference between older people and younger people occurs with sports associations, where young people are roughly 4.5 times more likely to be members than older people. Older people are also less frequently members of a trade union, educational association or organization with a community object. Naturally, this depends on the stage of life of the older person concerned; it is primarily people who are involved with education or participate in the labour market who are members of an educational association or trade union. Older people are more frequently members of a political party or women's association than people aged 35 to 54.

People in the 55 to 74 age group are more often members of a hobby, choral, music or amateur dramatic society than people aged under 55 or over 75. A distinction can be drawn between the organizations concerned mainly with furthering a certain interest (such as a political party or an organization with a community object) and associations that are of a more social nature (such as sports or hobby associations). People are significantly more frequently members of interest groups than social clubs. Membership rates decline with increasing age in both types of association, although this is most marked in social clubs. The differences among older people are in fact generally greater than the differences between the over-55s and the under-55s. The group of over-75s has the fewest members (SCP 1998: 149) and these are often 'paper' members.

Roughly a quarter of older people are members of an older people's association or senior citizens' council. Around 525,000 older people are currently members of one of the four national older people's associations. These associations promote the interests of older people and strive for their equal treatment in society. Between 1980 and 1997 the membership of these associations increased by 36 per cent; the total number of over-50s in society increased over the same period by 21 per cent. This means that the percentage of older people who are members of an older people's association has grown; in 1996–97, 12 per cent of people aged over 50 were members of such an association: in 1980 the figure was 11 per cent. Participation increased from 56 per cent to 63 per cent between 1983 and 1995. This increase occurs in all age categories, but is greatest among older people. In particular, the percentage of the over-75s who are members of an association has increased (by 75 per cent). Not only has the percentage of Dutch citizens who are members of an association risen considerably since the early 1990s, but people have also begun to combine memberships more frequently. In 1979, 24 per cent of people aged 35 to 54 were members of several associations; the figure in 1995 was 37 per cent. The proportion of older people aged 55 to 74 who are members of several associations increased over the same period from 16 per cent to 26 per cent (SCP 1996a: 541). A 1992 study by Statistics Netherlands (CBS) showed that 73 per cent of over-55s count themselves as members of a Church, whereas 56 per cent of these people (41 per cent of all older people) attend church at least once a month (SCP 1998: 151–4).

Voluntary work

Whether or not someone participates in voluntary work, as well as the number of voluntary activities that person performs, is related to age. In general, the older people are the less voluntary work they do: 50 to 64 year olds perform voluntary work slightly less frequently (approximately 62 per cent) than 35 to 49 year olds (66 per cent), but the differences are small. After age 65 participation in voluntary work declines and is especially low among the over-75s (26 per cent). As regards the number of voluntary activities a person carries out, it is striking that, compared with 50 to 59 year olds, 60 to 64 year olds perform several activities relatively frequently. In other words, the proportion of people who do voluntary work is no bigger in this group than in the younger age groups but those who perform voluntary work are more often active on several fronts. Roughly one-third of those aged under 75 provide informal help within their own network. Those aged 55 to 59 give informal help slightly more often than the other age groups; it may be that this group more often has a combination of small grandchildren and needy parents (SCP 1998).

The breakdown by gender shows that there is a (weak) correlation between age and participation in voluntary work for both men and women: although people participate less in voluntary work with increasing age there is an exception for women in the 55 to 59 age group; this is probably because, as mentioned earlier, members of this age group in particular provide a great deal of informal help within their own network; and women provide this type of help more often than men (De Klerk and Timmermans 1999: 162). Among the over-65s, by contrast, the proportion of men is higher than that of women. It may be that these people do a lot of administrative work, an activity that is carried out mainly by men, often in later life (De Klerk and Timmermans 1999: 158; SCP 2001: 52–3).

Leisure activities

Older people currently have a broader and less saturated pattern of leisure activity than they had 20 years ago, and they are much more likely to seek entertainment away from the home. Of course, differences remain between the various categories of older people. The higher their socio-economic status, the better their health and the younger they are, the more time they spend outside their home and the more diverse their pattern of activities. One striking point is that both religiosity and the availability of transport have a positive impact on the pattern of activities. Older people now spend much more time participating in sport than in the past, and they spend less time on domestic contacts. Within certain individual leisure activities, there has been a shift from pastimes for which no specific facilities are needed to specialized leisure activities in the leisure market (SCP 1996).

Loneliness and isolation

At the moment the most prevalent opinion in social science in the Netherlands is that loneliness means a lack *of* contacts or a lack *in* contacts (Linneman *et al.* 2001). Loneliness can be regarded as the discrepancy between what one wants in terms of interpersonal affection and intimacy and what one has; the greater the discrepancy, the greater the loneliness. The importance of social perceptions and evaluations of one's personal relationships is emphasized (De Jong Gierveld 1989). Three aspects are consistent: loneliness has to do with shortages in the social relations someone has, it is a feeling and is different from being alone, and it is unpleasant and dejecting (Linneman *et al.* 2001: 14). It occurs in each stage of life but increases with age (Linnemann 1996).

Estimates of the percentage of older people who suffer from a regular recurrence or stronger long-lasting forms of loneliness vary from 4 per cent to 22 per cent (RMO-advies 1997). De Jong Gierveld (1999) has developed, on the basis of empirical studies of loneliness among Dutch men and women, a set of norm scores. The scale consists of 11 items describing the presence or absence of a discrepancy between the social relations a person has and the social relations he or she wants. Scale scores range from 0, indicating the absence of loneliness feelings, to 11, indicating severe loneliness. Based on cutting scores of 3 (to distinguish between lonely people and not lonely people), 9 (between severely lonely or lonely people and others) and 11 (between severely lonely people and others), figures show that 68 per cent of the older people in the Netherlands are not lonely, 28 per cent are moderately lonely (score 3.0 to 8.0), 3 per cent are lonely (score 9.0 and 10.0) and 1 per cent are extremely lonely (score 11.0). The lowest average loneliness scores (1.0) were observed among older people living with a partner and having a large personal network.

The highest average loneliness scores (4.9) were observed among single divorced older people with a small network (De Jong Gierveld 1999).

Several researchers have focused on the relationship between the life situation and the extent of loneliness. The following tentative conclusions can be drawn. Older people with a partner are more likely to be happy and not to be lonely, than individuals without a partner (De Jong Gierveld and Van Tilburg 1995). The loss of a partner is one of the most important causes of loneliness (Dugan and Kivett 1994). Men without a partner are in general more lonely than women without a partner (Linneman *et al.* 2001). Socio-economic circumstances mainly have an indirect relationship with loneliness. Those with a higher education and a higher income have, in general, larger networks and are therefore less vulnerable to loneliness (Dykstra and Gierveld 1999). Having a relationship based on mutual trust plays a role. The presence of one or more people whom one can trust, such as a friend, siblings and so on, reduces the chances of feelings of loneliness. Living alone and having few contacts in the neighbourhood makes people more sensitive to loneliness (Linneman *et al.* 2001).

Loneliness appears not to be related to ageing *per se*, but rather to circumstances that change with age, such as the absence of a partner, a limited network, and a limited number of frequent contacts, as well as a poor health rating. The most lonely are not necessarily the oldest people but are those who have limited resources in terms of relationships and/or in terms of health (De Jong Gierveld and Van Tilburg 1995). Health, especially subjective health, has a direct effect on loneliness. Being in good health shapes the conditions for developing and maintaining involvement in mediating structures and poor health is directly associated with feelings of loneliness (Penninx 1994; Knipscheer *et al.* 1995).

Participation and policy

One of the objectives of Dutch policy on older people is to increase their participation in society. The question of whether this participation is adequate is, however, difficult to answer as there are no standards against which this can be measured – though to some extent such standards are implied in the constant comparison with the participation of 35 to 54 year olds. There is an implicit assumption here that older people ought to participate in the community just as much as the generation after them. If, for example, they have a lower income or a smaller home, or if they participate in sport less often, the conclusion is quickly drawn that older people are disadvantaged and that this demands a solution. In identifying differences between age categories, whether older people themselves perceive this as a problem is often ignored. It is impossible to avoid this because in general no data are available on the views of older people. In the few cases where those views are known, it turns out that older people sometimes experience the problems identified differently: older people less often participate in education and use computers less frequently, but when they are asked what they think, many of them turn out not to have any interest in these matters. Evidently they do not see themselves as disadvantaged in this respect. A large number of older people, particularly those of advanced age, will have no interest in participating in voluntary work. The question is whether the government should pursue policy in these areas for these people. On the one hand, both society and the older people concerned can benefit from an active older population; on the other hand, people have the individual freedom to decide how they wish to structure their lives (SCP 2001: 287–8).

Role of services in quality of life

The main care providers in the system of elder care are home care, residential homes and nursing homes. Older people in need of help or care mostly in the first instance apply to the local (or regional, for that matter) Home Care Organization, or to a GP or a community social service centre. These will refer the older person to a needs assessment agency for clarification of demand, assessment of need and allocation of kind and quantity of care.

Home care is the combination of home nursing and home help. Mostly home care delivery is integrated: most home care organizations offer both home nursing and home help. Formerly home nursing and home help used to be separate organizations. For years now there has been a process of integration and merging but occasionally there are still separate home-nursing and home-help organizations. Of course, even in the case where there are separate organizations, nursing and home help have to be integrated on the operational level; very often, a client who needs home nursing also needs home help. This requires intensive cooperation between the two organizations. Some clients who apply for home help may be given 'alpha help', which is a kind of household chores assistance done by housewives who are hired and paid by the client and for which the home-help organization is just an intermediary. As home-care organizations work locally (or regionally) they have their own catchment areas where they have almost no competition, apart from an occasional minor challenge by a commercial home-nursing organization (mostly in larger cities) and by some community activities of residential homes.

If older people who are dependent on care and help cannot cope any longer at home they may apply to be admitted to a residential home. (The literal translation of the Dutch word is 'caring home'.) Those admitted do not need special medical care or nursing (otherwise they might be referred to a nursing home). Consequently, there are hardly any qualified nurses among the staff; most of the employees are care staff with an intermediate or lower education. In principle, residents keep their own GPs. In case residents might develop dementia later on, attempts are generally made to keep them in a special care project rather than transferring them to a nursing home.

If individuals are in a stable situation but they are still not able to cope at home and need non-complex continuous care, they may be referred to a nursing home, which is for long-term care and nursing. There are three kinds of nursing homes. One is for the physically disabled, and one for psychogeriatric patients, mainly demented older people. The third kind of nursing home is a combination of these two. This is the most frequent kind and it has special wards for dementia patients. Nursing homes also have an important function in the more short-term rehabilitation of both older and younger patients and in diagnosis and functional assessment. Qualified medical, paramedical and nursing staff are present in nursing homes. Nursing-home medicine is a special discipline in the Netherlands, being a combination of geriatric, rehabilitation and GP competences.

Admission to home care, residential homes and nursing homes is subject to needs assessment. Whereas until 1998 home care did its own needs assessment, and assessment for institutional care was carried out by a separate agency, nowadays there are independent and integrated needs assessment agencies, which cover both home-care and institutional care admission. They are organized at the regional level, so they are called regional needs assessment agencies (RIOs). There is no nationwide protocol in use for assessment, but procedures used by RIOs are often based on the ICIDH. For assessment in cases of (suspected) dementia very often the regional community mental care organization (RIAGG) is enlisted, then a social geriatrician or a specialized psychologist might be involved. In the near future RIO will also be charged with the assessment of disabled persons.

Insurance

All citizens are eligible for the four types of care mentioned above in the framework of a general public long-term care insurance (AWBZ), which guarantees not so much access to care but rather financial compensation for officially permitted care suppliers and equity for the patients. Access to care is not subject to means or asset testing; however, patients, residents or clients will pay a (maximized) co-payment, the exact amount being income dependent. Providers are private not-for-profit organizations (with very few exceptions) but are funded in the framework of AWBZ. Hospitals are not under the rule of the care insurance but rather that of the health insurance. Hence, no needs assessment by RIO is required. Older patients whose condition is more complex, acute or uncertain, may be referred to a geriatric department of a hospital (GAAZ), which exist in all major hospitals. Also older patients with multiple morbidity may be admitted for diagnosis and therapy.

Recent developments in policy on care of older people

Due to the pressure of the gradually ageing population on the public purse and the 'independence ideal' of the young old, elder care has to modernize. Important themes in modernization are: accessibility, the spread of services, and appropriateness in the organization and implementation of care and provision of services. Government policy is aimed at encouraging independent living and a transition from institutionalized to semi-institutionalized and community-based provision. There is a marked reduction in scale in residential care homes, with the average number of beds/living units and residents being smaller; at the same time the amount of space per living unit has increased sharply in recent years (SER 1999; SCP 2001). Local authorities have been given more responsibility (for example, the Services for the Disabled Act; local authorities are responsible for the delivery of housing, transport services and wheelchairs). Since the end of the 1980s, welfare policy has been the responsibility of local authorities. The availability of welfare services and activities for older people is highly diverse and ranges from practical service delivery and reception to recreational activities and education. Little is known about the size of the supply, the takeup or costs of the welfare system for older people. Although no studies are available that demonstrate the effects of this service provision, it is undeniably the case that provisions such as the meals service, the personal alarm service and day care are important for a number of less self-reliant older people in enabling them to maintain their independence. The small amount of research that has been carried out appears to suggest that welfare provisions are subjectively indispensable for a small group of older people in making their lives more pleasant and enabling them to live independently (SCP 2001: 179–85). Independence is an ideal that is taken seriously in government services. This seems to meet the needs of older people who would like to arrange their own lives.

Client-linked budget: a new way of finance

The person-allocated or individualized budget is a new form of funding for healthcare. The person-allocated budget (PGB) is a sum of money provided to individuals with a particular requirement for care and who have a preference for money rather than the more normal help in kind. The person receiving the budget can spend the money as he or she sees fit. The idea behind the PGB is that people will then exert greater influence over the care they receive. Budgetholders are responsible for finding a suitable solution and choose a carer themselves and determine the nature, scale and content of the help as well as the conditions of employment. At this moment the use of the PGB is very small, but in the near future it will become much better known and more popular. Budgetholders are not alone in assessing the PGB positively; other parties involved with it (such as the Sickness Funds Council) regard the PGB as a valuable alternative to care in kind (Driest and Weekers 1998; Ramakers and Miltenburg 1998).

At present the PGB is possible only for people having a medical requirement for less than three hours a day of professional home care. The present State Secretary is considering an extension of the PGB by older people's home- and nursing-home care (Tweede Kamer 1998/1999); this would then mean that those with an indication for nursing-home or older people's home care and in need of a greater number of hours of professional care each day would also be able to make use of a PGB and so postpone or avoid admission if they so wished. It may be anticipated that as soon as there is an equivalent choice between a budget and care in kind, at least 40 per cent of people with a long-term dependence on home care will opt for a budget (Ramakers and Miltenburg 1998 in SCP 1998). Furthermore, PGB users are relatively young. Allowance would also need to be made for a limited suction effect (10 per cent) as a PGB would be better able to meet the needs of people with a medical condition who for various reasons did not regard care in kind as a solution and consequently did not make use of subsidized care.

The government continues to play an important role under a PGB system, especially as regards monitoring the quality of the nursing and care. In assessing the quality of household help, reliance must primarily be placed on the opinion of users themselves (SCP 1998: 129–36).

The use of care in care homes

Independence has become part of the lifestyle of the new generation of young older people (Timmermans *et al.* 1997a in SCP 2001). This emphasis on independence is reflected, for example, in the preference shown by older people for independent rather than institutionalized housing. Policy makers and care institutions are responding to this trend; whereas care for older people in the 1970s consisted primarily of older people's homes and home-help organizations (SCP 1998), today there is a wide range of provisions available for this age group. These provisions are aimed at preventing or compensating for limitations.

Two-thirds of older households living independently are able to manage without informal or private help or home care. There are various reasons for non-takeup: these people are relatively healthy; their living and residential situation means that they do not need to apply for help; or there is limited access to professional help. For a very small group of older people, the non-takeup of care provision is related to self-neglect (SCP 2001).

Earlier research has shown that 72 per cent of nursing home residents generally feel at home (De Veer and Kerkstra 1998). Residents of traditional care homes also express a positive view of living in the institution (Wever 2000); around 80 per cent of residents feel that sufficient help is provided, and the same percentage is satisfied with the quality of the help offered (SCP 2001: 211–12).

Little is known about the professional and informal care offered in institutions. The percentage of nursing-home residents receiving professional help with personal care, nursing treatments and mobility is high, as might be expected. Care-home residents are much more frequently self-reliant: roughly half receive professional help with nursing treatments, personal care or light household activities; almost 90 per cent require no help with mobility. Informal care also plays an important role in institutions. Roughly a third of nursing-home residents receive weekly help with mobility from informal helpers; a quarter of them receive help with personal care. This finding may point to a shortage of staff in nursing homes, for example, or to a greater need for care on the part of specific resident groups (SCP 1998).

Most older people in care and nursing homes and in sheltered housing have a religious conviction and see themselves as religious. Care-home residents are more often (very) religious than others. A majority of the religious residents of institutions consider it important to be able to talk to a spiritual carer – rather than with the institution staff – about life issues. In general, residents are satisfied regarding the time and attention they receive in this regard. Nevertheless there is a sizeable group – a quarter of religious residents of care homes and a fifth of nursing-home residents – who are dissatisfied with this aspect. More than a quarter of residents are also dissatisfied regarding the attention devoted to this subject by staff, an issue that is considered important by nursing-home patients in particular (SCP 2001).

Life satisfaction and subjective wellbeing

Physical health is one of the most important aspects of QoL: if people are healthy they will have a higher QoL than if they are suffering from health complaints. Another indicator of QoL is someone's wellbeing (the extent to which people consider themselves to be happy and satisfied with the life they are leading). Most people feel happy. This also applies to older people, although the percentage declines somewhat with age. Nearly half are satisfied with the lives they lead. Once again this percentage falls slightly with age.

Roughly a sixth are downright dissatisfied with life. People more often feel lonely or downcast as they grow older. By contrast older people less frequently feel out of sorts or restless than people aged under 55. Over 20 per cent of the over-75s suffer frequently or very frequently from the first of these complaints (feeling lonely or downcast) – roughly twice as many as people aged 35 to 54 (SCP 1998). People who feel less healthy score less well for all aspects of wellbeing than people who feel healthy. The type of household and gender also play a role. Single householders generally have a lower sense of wellbeing than cohabiting people and women often have a lower sense of wellbeing than men. After adjusting for the other factors, age does not affect wellbeing. In other words, the previously noted differences between people in various age categories are to a large extent caused by the fact that people suffer more frequently from health problems and more frequently live alone at more advanced ages (SCP 1998: 120–2).

Subjective assessments

Older people are inclined to assess their health more positively than would appear to be justified according to an 'objective' criterion such as medical opinion (Deeg and Hoeymans 1997 in SCP 2001: 117). At the end of the 1990s there were more people than in previous years who considered their health status to be moderate or poor, especially among women. It may be that a difference in the method of data gathering is responsible for this but it may also indicate higher ambitions of the population with regard to their health (Kronjee refers to this in Deeg *et al.* 2000). Comparison with the figures from the 1956 National Longitudinal Survey of the Elderly confirms this latter suspicion (Pot and Deeg 1997). People in the older age categories assess their health as poor more often than younger people but from the age of 75 onwards there is little further increase in the feeling of being unwell: slightly less than a fifth of the very old feel not very healthy. The Leiden-85+ study showed that 75 per cent of the very elderly living at home who were questioned – all aged 85 or more – assess their health as 'good' to 'very good' (Gussekloo *et al.* 2000).

Residents of sheltered housing or institutions assess their own health more negatively than older people living independently, as might be expected. These differences disappear for people aged 85 and over; this group assesses its own health as poor or moderate roughly just as often. Many older people label their health 'moderate'; the opinion 'poor' is given less often. Their opinions on their own health are evidently adapted to the circumstance of having less good health and may therefore present an overly favourable picture of the health status of the older population. But if that is the case, it can in any event be observed that health problems do not undermine the feeling of wellbeing of many older people, including a fairly large number of older people in institutions (SCP 2001: 117).

Limitations experienced by people in their daily lives as a result of health problems are often the result of physical impairments, although problems relating to stamina and in particular pain also have a major impact. Older people living in institutions report severe pain more frequently than those living independently. The very elderly living at home and in institutions differ little in their experience of pain, however: a relatively large number – one-third – of both groups experience (very) severe limitations through pain. With advancing age the number of older people living independently who suffer from severe pain increases.

Roughly a quarter of the population aged 35 and over feel at least slightly limited by chronic disorders or disabilities; 10 per cent feel severely limited. Among older people these percentages are generally a good deal higher: in 1999 a quarter of the oldest age group feel severely limited in their daily lives through health problems. Not everyone who experiences limitations is continually hindered by them. Around 10 to 20 per cent of people with an illness or disorder say that they rarely or never suffer limitations because of it. The same proportion occasionally experienced limitations. Roughly a quarter of older people living at home say they are continually hindered by their illness. This latter category increases in size with age: from 9 per cent among 35 to 54 year olds to 28 per cent for those aged 75 and over. The complaints and limitations do come and go, but increasingly remain in the oldest age groups (SCP 2001: 143–4).

Future research priorities

The Netherlands does have an extensive tradition of research on ageing but this has its limitations and does not answer all the questions of both researchers and policy makers.

For about five years a number of sectors/organizations in the care area have initiated some benchmarking research. That means they have been looking quite thoroughly at the outcomes of their work. It shows that they are growing more aware of the importance of quality of care. However, this does not mean that there is no need for special evaluation research in the strict sense. In order to be able to demonstrate the contribution of special services, (policy) programmes or planned social activities, a research programme based on a real field experimental design is needed. This type of research is hardly seen in the Netherlands. Convincing evidence will be needed in the next decades in order to argue for the future investments in elder programmes and care.

A second area that needs particular attention is an integrated approach to the living environment. It should take into account all the aspects of the living environment: accessibility of houses and public buildings, safety on the street (think of traffic, crime, falls), composition of the populations, availability of shops nearby, neighbourhood centres, care services. The need for a strategic approach to housing and living arrangements for older people will increase over future decades; on the one hand, because of the increasing number of older people in most Western countries and, on the other hand, also because there appears to be an increasing resistance to living in a residential home. Dutch policy is clearly moving in the direction of constructing live-and-care zones within the community. This asks for a integrative approach to independent living within the community in close connection with availability of services.

A third topic for future research is related to migration and ageing. Different ethnic minority groups are rapidly growing older in the Netherlands. Members of these groups seem to be particularly vulnerable, due to their socio-economic status – low labour market participation, low income and so on – and their poor command of the Dutch language. They are facing more problems and have few resources to solve these problems. Because of their vulnerability they constitute important target groups for policy on older people in the Netherlands. In order to introduce good policy for older people from ethnic minorities, information about their life situation, position, needs and demands is of crucial importance. At this moment the information is not at hand or complete. Further mapping out of the living arrangements and needs of ethnic minorities in a broad study is important in order to provide and maintain a high QoL for them.

Conclusion

The Netherlands has a strong tradition of social network research among older people, which reflects awareness of the importance of interpersonal relationships to QoL in old age. A recent focus of policy has been on the prevention of loneliness but there is some reluctance on the part of the Dutch government to push its policy on social participation too strongly. Non-governmental organizations representing older people could play a key role but they are largely absent from policy discussions on this issue. However, the government does have access to evidence about conditions in old age through its regular surveys of wellbeing in the population as a whole. Also there are many examples which illustrate the inventiveness shown by Dutch society in responding to its own ageing.

Note

1. The Nestor study was a national cross-sectional study conducted in 1992 among people aged 55–85 (n = 4500), which focussed on social networks and lifecourse data. The Longitudinal Ageing Study Amsterdam (LASA) built on NESTOR with a longitudinal study of the social, cognitive, emotional and physical dimensions of ageing. The fourth round of observation was undertaken in 2002. (Deeg and Westendorp-de Seriere 1994; Deeg *et al.* 1998; http: //www.ssg.scw.vu.nl/lasa)

2. The Time Use Survey (TBO) is held among the Dutch population once every five years. In addition to background questions, general questions are asked about how people spend their time. Respondents are asked to keep a diary for a one-week period, entering the activities on which each quarter of an hour is spent.

10

Sweden: quality of life in old age II

Lars Andersson

Family and support networks

In order to analyse the extent of networks it is necessary to identify who are included in what the individual regards as family and, specifically, the place of elderly parents. In 1989 a simple random sample of Swedes aged 20 to 59 was asked to describe what they regarded as their family. In conclusion, only the constellation 'mother, father, child/children who share household' is considered by all to be a family (Trost 1993). Apart from that definitions are disparate (Andersson and Sundström 1996). Trost (1993) identifies three psychological factors that determine whether someone will be included in the individual's family – emotional closeness, fairness, and caring responsibility.

With every new generation the multiplicity of family and co-residence arrangements increases, and the relative size of the different groups changes. Since the mid-1980s, for example, the number of divorcees has increasingly exceeded the number of widows/widowers in the 60 to 65 age group and is now more than double the number (SOU 2002: 29).

As for older people, there are now mainly two options in Sweden: married/ cohabiting or living alone. Both lifestyles have become more common in the past decades. During the 1980s and 1990s the proportion of people aged 65 years and above who were cohabiting in one form or another increased, particularly among older men. However, one in three of both sexes aged 65 to 74 lives alone and likewise half of those aged 75 to 84. In the latter age group, the number of women living alone is nearly double that of men, 65 per cent compared with 31 per cent (SOU 2002: 29; Statistics Sweden 2000).

There are also some signs of an increase among the young old in couples who maintain two separate households. While young-old men still prefer to establish conventional relationships, young-old women are becoming more prone to try out new forms of relationships without the commitments typical for marriage. For young-old women it can be important to keep their own apartment in order to balance the needs for intimacy and seclusion. This living apart can also function as a protection against the expectation of eventually becoming an informal carer. The chances for a man to receive public home help are reduced if there is a woman in the household (SOU 2002: 29).

Households are becoming smaller for all age groups. From a 'traditional' level of about 10 per cent who lived alone, this increased to 39 per cent in 1988–89 (men 24 per cent, women 50 per cent). According to the Eurobarometer, from 1992/93 (Andersson 1993) close to four out of ten Swedes aged 60 and over lived in single households, and about 60 per cent belonged to a two-person household. Other living arrangements, such as living with offspring, siblings or others, or living in institutions, have vanished or shrunk considerably (Andersson and Sundström 1996). According to the Eurobarometer only 3 per cent belonged to a household of more than two persons.

In 1954, 27 per cent of older people in Sweden lived with one or more offspring, in 1975 the corresponding figure was 9 per cent; today it is a mere 2 per cent. There are hardly any grandchildren present in the households of older people today, and they have never been very frequent. The offspring who moved out did not move very far. The majority of older people (63 per cent) have a child living within 15 km, which is a proportion near to that reported from other countries (Andersson and Sundström 1996).

At the end of the 1990s about 53 per cent of the 65 to 84 age group met with their children at least once a week. About 30 per cent did not have a close friend outside the household or family, a decrease of about 8 per cent in 15 years. About 3 per cent of those aged 75 to 84, and 1.7 per cent among the 65 to 74 year olds are estimated to have limited social relationships – that is they meet people outside their own households at most a few times per year. The last two figures were twice as high 15 years earlier (Statistics Sweden, 2000). There is no evidence that the social relationships among generations in the family would decrease. Data on generational relationships in general are lacking.

Solitary householding will not increase any more, but when we talk about living alone in old age what we really should think about is the risk rather than the average prevalence. The risk of eventually living alone and dying in that situation is of course much higher than suggested by the average rate as both parties in a couple usually do not die simultaneously. Swedish longitudinal data indicate that some 70 per cent of older women will live alone during the last part of their life, as compared to 30 per cent of the men (Andersson and Sundström 1996).

Living alone is often portrayed as being tantamount to isolation and loneliness. However, despite the large proportion of solitary households, older people in Sweden come first in all network relevant measures in a 13-country comparison (the 12 EU countries in 1992 plus Sweden in 1993). They have the third highest figure (after Denmark and Ireland) for contacts with family during the previous week (73.4 per cent), and the second highest figure (after Ireland) for contacts with friends (70.1 per cent). Older people in Sweden come out first in contacts with young people, and their perceptions of the extended network is the most positive in nine out of 11 cases. In addition, the percentage who often feel lonely (6 per cent), is the second lowest (after Denmark).

Despite a considerable amount of research in the field of family and support networks, we have little knowledge of the importance of socio-economic factors – how different living conditions and ways of living affect approaches and opportunities to provide assistance and support to older people and willingness to do so. A study by Winqvist (1999) focuses on the societal context of these issues and the aim is to understand the relationship between the life mode and the approach of adult children towards a parent in need of care or assistance.

The point of departure was the life mode theory, which includes the different life modes of the self-employed person, the wage earner and the careerist. The three life modes can be described as representing three different cultures where each one has its own ideological conceptual context. The situation of the self-employed person is undifferentiated in the sense that there are no definite borders between work and leisure. For the wage earner, the relationship between work and leisure is characterized by a means-goal approach. The careerist, on the other hand, lives in order to work. The life modes are theoretical concepts and may be mixed.

The approach of the *self-employed* person towards his/her parent is referred to as *an integrated matter of course*. This involves an unreflecting approach to contact with the parent, where that which needs to be done is done without giving it much thought. The approach of the *wage earner* is referred to as *a matter of family loyalty*, where the inherent value of being of assistance and keeping the family together is emphasized. The approach of the *careerist*, referred to as *a competing circumstance*, does not allow for the parent playing a 'natural' part in the everyday life of the adult child. The three approaches are referred to in terms of ideal types.

The ideal typical understanding of the self-employed person can be described in terms of the relationship to the parent being an inherent part of everyday life. Contact with the parent is frequent. Providing assistance is understood as a 'natural' part of everyday life and the obligations of adult children are understood in terms of personal responsibility. This does not mean, however, that the self-employed person views this responsibility as a burden. Social contact with the parent is oriented towards performing certain practical tasks. Assisting the parent is a way of socializing. It is quite acceptable for the adult child to live close by, but not to live with the parent. As assistance is an inherent part of everyday life, the need for municipal home help only applies when the parent's need for assistance is substantial.

For the wage earner all social contact with the parent has to take place during free time. Contact is frequent and meets with the criteria for good leisure: it is meaningful and pleasant. This can be described as an altruistic approach. The children are prepared to help the parent with that which needs to be done, but the fixed hours at work are restrictive and if the siblings cannot satisfy the parent's need for assistance, municipal home help is used. Living together with the parent is a possibility and providing assistance is motivated in terms of caring for and loving the parent.

For the careerist work takes a lot of time and effort, which means that it is difficult to spend much time with the parent. If the careerist does not decide a time for meeting the parent on a regular basis, it is unlikely that a meeting takes place at all. Careerists cannot imagine changing their working hours for the sake of the parent and they prefer not to live too close to the parent. Living with the parent is out of the question. The careerist does not spend a lot of time providing assistance on a regular basis. These kinds of tasks are carried out by siblings, when there are any, who represent other life modes, and by paid staff. One motive for providing assistance is partly selfish: it brings about a feeling of satisfaction. A feeling of imbalance in the relationship is experienced when the careerist feels the burden from the emotional dependence of the parent and from not receiving a lot out of the social contact. This can result in the careerist feeling guilty.

Participation and activity

There are more-or-less explicit age norms that govern the participation and influence of older people in society. These norms imply a withdrawal at approximately age 65 to 70. In addition, claims for intensifying and regenerating democracy and citizenship are often accompanied by demands for increased participation of younger people.

A recent governmental democracy committee has noted that older people are underrepresented among elected representatives, but does not discuss the political influence of older people. In accordance with its directives it discusses women, children and young people, immigrants and handicapped people (SOU 2002: 29). The government bill on democracy, based on the report from the democracy committee, does make a reference to the political participation of older people. However, when long-term goals are considered, there is no mention of increased participation by older people. Instead, it is stated that the participation of young people, unemployed, and immigrants should increase (SOU 2002: 29).

The official retirement age of 65 with regard to work is also valid for representative positions, held on behalf of political parties or societies, on management boards known as political 'commissions of trust', which decline markedly beyond 66. The overrepresentation of individuals aged 60 to 66 on such committees (Table 10.1) makes the change in participation rate even more obvious. The same change can be seen for members of the boards in Swedish PLCs (Figure 10.1).

With respect to civic activities, almost 60 per cent of men aged 65 to 84 have on some occasion spoken at a meeting. The corresponding figure for women is half of that. The same proportion applies for contacting a civil servant (men 31 per cent, women 14 per cent). However, about one-third of both men and women have signed a petition. For participation in elections, the highest figures can be found in the age group 65 to 74, whereas among those aged 75 and above the figure is even lower than among first-time voters (SOU 2002: 29).

Table 10.1 Municipal commissions of trust compared to the share of the electorate for various age groups (%)

Age	Commissions of trust	Electorate	Difference
18–29	6	19	−13
30–44	24	27	−3
45–59	32	26	+6
60–6	31	8	+23
67+	7	20	−13

Source: SOU (2002: 29).

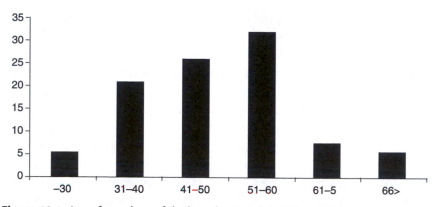

Figure 10.1 Age of members of the board in Swedish PLCs in 2001.
Source: SOU (2002: 29).

In 2000, about 88 per cent of men and 82 per cent of women aged 65 to 84 were members of an organization, and 40 per cent of men and 33 per cent of women were active members. Twenty-three per cent of men and 17 per cent of women held representative positions on management boards or 'commissions of trust' (Table 10.2). These are fairly high figures for membership, and one reason is the high membership of pensioners' organizations. Older people also have an influential position in disability and patient organizations. There are also many older members in sports organizations, motor organizations

Table 10.2 Social activities (%)

	Commissions of trust		Active member of a society/club		Member of a society/club	
	1992	2000	1992	2000	1992	2000
Total	**28.7**	**26.9**	**52.3**	**44.2**	**92.2**	**90.2**
Men						
45–64	40.4	36.2	57.4	51.5	95.4	95.1
65–84	26.2	22.6	40.6	40.3	88.0	88.2
Women						
45–64	28.8	27.9	47.9	42.2	96.0	95.2
65–84	12.0	17.0	35.7	32.8	81.8	82.4

Source: SOU (2002: 29).

(mostly males), housing organizations, religious organizations, consumers' co-operatives, humanitarian relief organizations, and organizations for culture, music or theatre. According to a study from 1998, 22 per cent in the age group 60 to 74 had engaged in voluntary work at some point during the previous year (SOU 2002 : 29).

Thus, older people are important as active members in many organizations that also attract younger people. Still, the contributions of older people are often associated with work for other older people based on age solidarity (SOU 2002: 29). The image of what constitutes successful ageing is heavily influenced by the views of important participants in the field. Jönson (2001) studied images of ageing and older people in the magazines of Sweden's two largest pensioner organizations – Pensionärernas Riksorganisation (PRO) with 380,000 members and Sveriges Pensionärsförbund (SPF) with 208,000 members. The research concluded that images of ageing in general have been affected by two stereotypes. One stereotype has described healthy, vital, and happy ageing while the other has focused on weakness, dependency and misery. In the magazines of the pensioner organizations, images of old age and older people have been ambiguous. Since the 1950s descriptions have celebrated characteristics that are typically associated with younger ages, such as strength and independence. On the other hand, the organizations have emphasized injustices and risks in old age, and thus have contributed to an overall image of older people as victims and a risk group. Furthermore, the two magazines' descriptions of older people and their position in society have differed during the same periods, and seem to have reflected ideological beliefs about the development of society. In that sense images of old age have expressed tensions and developments in the political landscape of Sweden (Jönson 2001). Why have the organizations and their magazines concentrated so strongly on images that express injustice and risks? Jönson's answer is that the organizations should be viewed as social movements that have to produce injustice and risk in order to mobilize members for collective action and make claims for social change. This approach involves a risk of stigmatizing older people, and the resulting low self-image could influence their QoL.

The role of services in quality of life

Although only a minority of older people are dependent on social services, the functioning of the social services is very important for those who need them.

There are two pieces of legislation which govern old age care: the Social Services Act of 1 January 2002 (SoL 2001: 453) and the Health and Medical Services Act of 1983. The responsibility is divided between three levels of government – the state, the county councils, and the municipalities.

The state sets out policy directives by means of legislation and economic steering measures. The county councils are responsible for the provision of healthcare, and the municipalities for social service and housing for older people (Johansson 2000). Both the county councils and the municipalities have the right to levy taxes.

Both healthcare and social services are subsidized. The recipients usually pay only a fraction of the actual cost, which varies among the municipalities. The total cost of care and services for the elderly in 1998 was estimated to make up about 6.5 per cent of GDP. Two-thirds of the cost goes to institutional care and one-third to outpatient healthcare and home help (Johansson 2000). Public expenditure for old age care has increased continuously, while the expenditure per person aged 80 and over has been relatively stable over time.

There is a statutory right to claim services and care, but each municipality decides its eligibility criteria and the range and level of services to be provided to those eligible. Determination of need takes place through a process of needs assessment carried out by a municipal care manager (sometimes by interdisciplinary care planning teams). If the person requesting services is dissatisfied with the decision, the case can be appealed in an administrative court (Johansson 2000).

The high percentage of women in the labour market (70 per cent), the fact that only about 2 per cent cohabit with children, and that there are no statutory requirements for children to provide care for their parents, presupposes a formal system of care for older people. With respect to informal care, the percentage of people receiving help from a spouse – in Sweden 32 per cent according to the Eurobarometer (Andersson 1993) – is the same as the average in the EU. The major difference between the countries is found in the percentage of help received from adult children who share a household with a frail older person. As noted above, coresidence with offspring is next to non-existent in Sweden. Consequently help from coresident children is rare (Andersson and Sundström 1996).

The most central of the services for older people is the home help. There are also other services such as transportation services, podiatry, meals on wheels, security alarms, home adaptations, handicap aids. In 1999 about 8 per cent of people aged 65 and over received home help. One-third of these also received home nursing care. In the 80 and over age group about one in five received home help (Table 10.3). The number of people receiving home help has reduced in relation to population growth since the late 1970s. However, the hours of help have increased – fewer persons receive help, but they receive more. Home help has, for example, to a larger extent been made available during weekends, evenings, and night hours. In 1988, 16 per cent of the recipients received help in the evenings and at night; the corresponding percentage in 1997 was 28. On average, the recipients receive 7 to 8 hours per week (Johansson 2000).

Table 10.3 Percentage of people with home help in ordinary housing, 2000

Age	Men	Women	Total
65–74	2.0	2.6	2.4
75–9	5.0	7.5	6.4
80–4	10.0	15.6	13.4
85–9	18.2	26.0	23.4
90+	27.6	31.9	30.8
Total	5.7	10.0	8.2
Total 80+	14.2	21.6	19.0

Source: SOU (2002: 29)

The development of institutional care is somewhat similar to home help. Until the early 1980s institutional care expanded in step with increases in the older population. Since then, the expansion has stagnated. In 1999 about 7.5 per cent of people aged 65 and over lived in institutions (the concept 'institutions' covers nursing homes, old age homes, service houses, group homes and so on). For people aged 80 and over the corresponding number was 20 per cent (Johansson 2000).

The availability of care varies over the country. The proportion of people aged 80 and over who receive home help has been shown to vary from 17 per cent in one municipality to 80 per cent in another, while the utilization of institutional care varied from 9 to 37 per cent. There is no evidence for a low percentage of home help being compensated for by a high level of institutionalization or the other way around (Trydegård 2000; Trydegård and Thorslund 2001, 2002).

The objective of the study by Trydegård (2000) was to describe and analyse the development of old age care in Sweden from a variety of perspectives and she found few obvious differences between different forms of care in terms of needs and use of care (Trydegård 1998). Home-based and institution-based care, for example, are not necessarily two extremes of a care chain. The majority of residents in the traditional forms of institution reported good or fairly good health in roughly the same proportion as those living in their own homes and receiving extensive home help – that is, high levels of care in home-help services and fairly low levels in some of the institutions. How could this be interpreted? To what extent is it a sign of a conscious policy on the part of the municipalities to take older people's choice and self-determination into consideration? Some older people definitely want to 'age at home' irrespective of their care needs, while others, even with very low levels of needs, want to move to the safety of sheltered housing. A different interpretation is that there is inadequate care planning of individual cases, with some care recipients receiving too little care and supervision and others receiving too much. In the former case, the implications for the individual are serious; in the latter, the economic implications for the municipalities are considerable.

Public old age care in Sweden has had a changing and dramatic development. Having originally been a restricted, chiefly institution-based, poor relief measure for the very needy, public old age care became universal and, at its peak in the late 1970s, reached about two-thirds of the population aged 80 and over. As mentioned above, the period since the mid-1980s has seen a considerable decline, and old age care today is again restricted, not to the poorest, but to very frail older people. Among those who are outside the formal care system, Szebehely (1999) traces an increasing dualization of the care they receive: market solutions for the better off and increased family care for the less well off.

Trydegård (2001, 2002) concludes that there is no homogeneous 'Swedish model' of old age care. The coverage and the formation of services – whether home based or institution based – varies considerably between municipalities. Only a small part of these variations can be explained by local structural or political factors. It seems more appropriate to talk about 'welfare municipalities' than one uniform welfare state.

Trydegård (2002) also notes that the local variations have a long history in Sweden and are linked to a tradition of strong local autonomy. When it comes to home-help coverage, past municipal traditions seem to have a greater influence than present conditions. There seems to be a path dependency in the sense that established traditions and earlier municipal policies influence the present supply of old-age care, even in the home-help services that do not have the inertia of buildings or other fixed assets. Thus, it should be emphasized that these differences are not dependent on the position of the municipality along the rich/poor or urban/rural continua; the possibility of receiving care, and a particular kind of care, is dependent on where in the country the person lives.

Life satisfaction and wellbeing

Quality of life in old age is not just influenced by the present situation. Öberg's study from 1997 gives examples of how the life lived is reflected in old age. The study is based on biographical interviews with Finns from the generation of 'the wars and the depression' (born 1905–15). Its central objective is to identify the ways of life or life strategies that end up in either a successful or a problematic old age. Biographical research has created a new and less stereotyped understanding of ageing. With its emphasis on viewing ageing as a process as opposed to a stage, biographical research has also shown that the meaning of old age cannot be separated from the rest of the lifecourse. The sample consisted of 37 urban people – 23 women and 14 men – aged 73 to 83 living in Helsinki. Previously married or single retirees were chosen, because of the interest in studying how an ageing individual copes with life without a spouse.

Six different ways of life are identified in the typology. Two ways of life, *the bitter life* and *life as a trapping pit*, end up in a problematic old age. The other four, *life as a hurdle race, the devoted silenced life, life as a job career* and *the sweet life*, describe different strategies for successful ageing. The identified ways of life did not follow any strict social class or gender boundaries, even though some central trends were found.

The connection between biography and society is particularly present in *life as a hurdle race*. For these informants the rural living conditions in childhood formed both their present value structures and their life world. Socio-historical events such as the execution of a father in the Civil War, the absence or death of a spouse during the wars, the evacuation of the family to other parts of the country, or severe economic problems also played a role in this way of life. *Life as a hurdle race* is characterized by the coping strategy specific for this generation: 'coping through repression'. The odds were against them, but as heroes in their own lives they fought and won the battle. In the light of the fact that good health in old age seems to be a prerequisite for successful ageing, the fact that these informants have undergone and overcome occasional periods of illness was one sign of their regaining of control over life in old age. Turning points such as divorce or widowhood, considered in gerontological research to be stressful transitions, actually turned out to be positive transitions in this way of life. It was found that it was only in the ways of life that end up in a problematic old age (*the bitter life*, and *life as a trapping pit*) that evidence of retirement shock was found. It was therefore concluded that it is not retirement *per se* that is the key to understanding a traumatic experience of retirement.

In a study by Trossholmen (2000) 'lifecourse' stories were used to interpret and understand the informants' (12 older women) view of a pensioner life. These women were retired and they had been gainfully employed during the greater part of their lives. At the time of the interviews, they all were, or had been, married and had at least one child. All of them were healthy and were still living in their own homes. Half of them were born in wealthy middle-class homes and half in poor working-class families. The middle-class informants were safely brought up and were rigorously controlled. Good and proper education was important and there were many rules. The working-class informants describe humiliation and condescending treatment from teachers at school as well as from the surrounding society. In both groups, they were expected to marry and have children. Being a housewife was even desirable for them as young girls. Eventually, however, they all entered the labour market.

The middle-class women think that most of the class distinctions have disappeared. They sometimes complain of a lack of appreciation from the younger generation. Some of them wish that their children had more time for them and were not so occupied with their careers. For the working-class women life has been a successful journey in many ways. Although they believe that class distinctions remain, they consider that everything is so much better now than during their childhood. The society and the younger generation treat them with respect and they feel that they have good relationships with their children, who, often highly educated, lead their own lives without any interference from their mothers.

Wellbeing in nonagenarians

Hillerås *et al.* (1998, 1999, 2000, 2001) has looked at the wellbeing of nonagenarians. Factors believed to influence three components of wellbeing – life satisfaction, positive affect, and negative affect – were examined. The study also examined activity patterns, factors related to activity, and the relationship between different types of activity and wellbeing. The subjects (n = 105) were 90 years and older, and scored 24 points or more on the MMSE. Life satisfaction was slightly lower than usually found in studies of young olds. Not surprisingly, respondents tended to have higher life satisfaction if they had excellent subjective health, good social relationships, participated in pleasurable activities, and if they were extraverted and had an emotionally stable personality.

The results also suggested that 'outlook on life', 'social and emotional ties', 'engagement with the outside world' and 'physical capability' are important contributors to subjective wellbeing. Generally, personality emerged as the major determinant of wellbeing. The situation for the nonagenarians may look quite satisfactory. However, the group that it is possible for researchers to interview is a highly selective one. In this study, they made up about one third of the original sample of nonagenarians.

Future research priorities

Much of the diversity found among older people can be described in relation to the social inequalities prevalent in society. The pathways to these inequalities are complex: previous occupational exposure certainly plays a role, as well as access to and use of healthcare, lifestyle and health behaviour, housing, leisure activities, and the ability or motivation to use information. The analysis of social class differences is an initial step in understanding diversity among older people. Exploring the influence of social class among older people offers the opportunity to understand further the cumulative effects of social class over the lifecourse.

Family issues are a central concern for gerontological research. The changes in family structure resulting from divorce, remarriage and fertility patterns have not been sufficiently studied. Research on normative family issues such as older peoples' social construction of family membership is important for our understanding of caring and support.

Much of the research on adjustment to retirement has concentrated on the individual in isolation and has failed to take account of family circumstances and relationships. The change from work life to retirement can affect marital relationships in various ways. Factors such as emotional quality of the relationship, and the conflict between spending time together and the loss of personal space have to be taken into consideration. Research on how families negotiate the transition from work to retirement is also of importance for the understanding of future economic standards and social life.

Conclusion

Older people contribute quite substantially to society in spite of age norms that 'expect' a withdrawal at approximately age 65 to 70.

Generally speaking, older Swedes are either married/cohabiting or live alone. Both lifestyles have become more common in the past decades, but the solitary household appears to have reached a plateau. Although the number of divorcees in the 60 to 65 age group has increased, it has been offset by a much lower number of widows and widowers. Cohabiting without being married has also become more common as well as, to a lesser extent, living together and maintaining separate households (LAT). The risk of eventually living alone is much higher than suggested by the average rate, as both parties in a couple usually do not die simultaneously.

Generally, the availability of care varies over the country to the extent that it seems more appropriate to talk about 'welfare communities' rather than one uniform welfare state.

11

The UK: quality of life in old age II

Alan Walker and Carol Walker

Family and support networks

One of the main themes underpinning a good quality of life identified by older people themselves is 'having good social relationships with family, friends, and neighbours' (Bowling *et al.* 2003). The reduction in social networks experienced by ethnic minority people following migration to the UK seems to lead people in such groups to place greater reliance on family contacts than is the case for the white population (Nazroo *et al.* 2003). With greater longevity there is an increasing proportion of families spanning two, three or more generations (Lago 2000). Nearly everyone in Great Britain has a living parent or child, and many have both. One-third of women born in 1930 still have mothers living when they reach the age of 60. However, major cultural and social changes, especially increased geographical mobility and migration and increased family breakdown, mean that intergenerational relationships, roles and expectations are changing (Hagestad 1985). While the role of the family is still central in older people's lives, it differs to that reported in earlier sociological studies such as by Townsend (1959).

Older people interviewed for the 2002 English Longitudinal Study of Ageing (ELSA) (Marmot *et al.* 2003) reported frequent contact with their children. More than half the older people interviewed saw their children at least once a week and more than 80 per cent of men and over 90 per cent of women spoke to one of their children on the telephone. Friends were also found to be an important part of both older men and women's social networks, regardless of age. More than half said that they met up with friends at least once a week, with women again having slightly higher levels of such contact. Contact with other family members is lower than that with children or friends but there is still frequent telephone contact: 61 per cent of women and 45 per cent of men had telephone contact with other relatives at least once a week. Contact is lower among older people who are still in the labour market. Frequency of personal contact decreases and letter/email contact increases as social class rises, which the researchers suggest might reflect the higher levels of mobility among professional and managerial classes.

Grandparenthood

With increased longevity more people are experiencing a grandparent/ grandchild relationship. However, the nature of the relationship today is much more diverse and complex than in the past. The GO research project conduct- ed by Clarke and Roberts (2003) confirmed the heterogeneity of grandparents' families and roles. The youngest grandparent interviewed was 37 and the oldest 94. The maximum number of grandchildren was 23. The increased incidence of family change, including relationship breakdown and remarriage, is having a significant impact on grandparents, grandchildren and family patterns. Over one-third of grandparents (38 per cent) had grandchildren in non-intact families and one-fifth (21 per cent) had step-grandchildren – more among grandparents under 70. One-third of the grandparents interviewed were under the age of 60; the majority of these were working. This inevitably has an impact on the nature of the relationship and the contact between grandparents and grandchildren.

Research by Clarke and Roberts (2003) stressed the continuing importance to grandparents of their relationship with their grandchildren. Grandparents interviewed for the study were unanimous in this view. Most rated the relationship with their grandchildren as 'one of the most important in my life'; over half (55 per cent) said that being a grandparent contributed 'enormously' to their quality of life and a third (31 per cent) said it contributed 'a lot'. Only 4 per cent said it contributed 'not at all'.

> The main feeling was of strong emotional closeness and the contribution grand- children made to the quality of their lives. The symbolic value of grandchildren was clearly important. They represented a sense of continuity and immortality. (Clarke and Roberts 2003: 1)

Contact with grandchildren could be quite frequent: three in five saw at least one grandchild every week. Forty per cent of grandparents wanted more contact with their grandchildren, 50 per cent said they had the right amount of contact and only 1 per cent said they wanted less contact. Proximity is obviously an important factor in frequency of contact. However, this factor may in some cases be engineered by family members moving nearer or further away from grandparents. The telephone, email and webcams provide increased opportunities for people to keep in close contact even when living far apart. Clarke and Roberts (2003) found that lineage was a more important factor than geography: paternal grandparents see less of their sons' children, especially if there is a family breakup. Wenger and Burholt's (2001) longitudinal study in rural Wales revealed that grandparents had more frequent contact with their grandchildren when the children were young. While 50 per cent of grandparents saw one of their grandchildren at least once a week and most at least once a month when the first wave was conducted in 1979, this had fallen to 25 per cent by 1999 when most of the grandchildren had grown into adulthood.

Grandparents play different roles in the lives of their children and grandchildren. The GO research identified three main types of support: practical, financial and emotional. Grandparents, particularly grandmothers, played a key role in childcare and are 'routinely used for practical support in times of normal upheaval like the arrival of new babies, moving house and illness of parent, but they also took a key role in more protracted crises (Clarke and Roberts 2003 : 2). Sixty per cent of grandparents looked after grandchildren under 15 years old and 54 per cent babysat. The researchers reported that some grandparents felt obliged to provide much more help with childcare than they would wish in order to help working daughters or daughters-in-law or when their children separated from their partners. Sixty-four per cent gave their grandchildren money. This was most likely among older grandparents, those with more grandchildren, those with young grandchildren and those with higher incomes. Grandparents often provided financial assistance following divorce or separation. The grandparent/grandchild relationship is a reciprocal one. Wenger and Burholt (2001) found that adult grandchildren tended to visit and stay more frequently after a grandparent had lost his or her spouse. In such circumstances they often provided the surviving grandparent with practical help, such as mowing the lawn, cutting wood or providing transport. As grandparents aged, grandchildren showed concern about their ability to cope.

Siblings

Wellbeing in later life is enhanced by good sibling relationships (Cicirelli 1988; Avioli 1989), which themselves have often been found to strengthen in later life

(Moyer 1992; Jerrome 1994a; Wenger and Burholt 1998). Closeness of the bond between siblings has been correlated with lower levels of depression in both men and women (Connidis 1989). Levels of functional support are less significant than the high level of affectional solidarity that exists. Relationships between siblings are particularly important for those older people who have no children. In the later years of life siblings are the only people who share family memories of parents and childhood. Sibling relationships are influenced by social network structure, geographical proximity, health and gender. The most intimate of sibling relationships has been found to be between sisters (Wilson *et al.* 1994).

Research into the closeness both of sibling relationships and parent-and-child relationships in old age found that, in 1979, one-third of child-parent relationships were loose knit and three-quarters of sibling relationships were loose knit but, by 1995, there had been an 18 per cent increase in loose knit relationships between children and parents, whereas loose knit sibling relationships had decreased by 15 per cent (Burholt and Wenger 1998). This indicates that the differences in solidarity in sibling or child-parent relationships had almost disappeared; both were divided more equally between loose knit and close knit relationships. In 1979 only 13 per cent of mothers received help from their children compared with 44 per cent in 1995 (Burholt and Wenger 1998).

Participation and activity

Research by the Institute for Volunteering found that people over the age of 60 comprised 44 per cent of volunteers. They work in a range of areas including the environment, heritage projects, education and social welfare. Most older volunteers are from middle-class occupational backgrounds, but many working-class people are successfully involved in welfare related activities. Table 11.1, which is drawn from the 2002 ELSA study, shows healthy levels of participation in voluntary work among both older men and women. Between the ages of 60 and 80 more than one person in ten does voluntary work of one sort or another. Virtually all of the volunteers (90 per cent) in the Institute for Volunteering study enjoyed what they were doing and thought it was worth while. Three-quarters wanted to continue volunteering for as long as possible only stopping when they had to.

The ELSA study (Marmot *et al.* 2003) shows that the proportions of older people who are members of an organization vary by age, sex and type of

Table 11.1 Older people involved in voluntary work, by age and gender (%)

	Men	Women
50–4	8.7	9.1
55–9	8.5	13.3
60–4	10.3	16.6
65–9	12.9	17.0
70–4	13.9	13.5
75–9	11.5	12.9
80+	7.2	6.2

Source: Marmot *et al.* (2003), Table 4A.2.

organization. Men and women above their respective retirement ages are less likely than younger people to belong to a political party, trade union or environmental group. Men are more likely than women to belong to such organizations. Older people of all ages are more likely to belong to a tenants' or other neighbourhood organization, and a Church or other religious organization. Women are more likely to belong to a charitable organization than men. Those in poorer health are less likely to be members of any organization.

The majority of both men and women in the ELSA sample are a member of at least one organization, 37.2 per cent of men and 41.5 per cent of women are not. There is a fall in organization membership as people age. This may be because of failing health or difficulty in getting to the location but it also could reflect the looser ties of older people to organizational activity.

The ELSA study also provides information on social and civic participation (Table 11.2) and cultural activities, which are discussed later. Voting rates are very high compared with the national average; they are slightly higher for men than women and tend to increase with age. Use of the Internet, email and mobile phones is much higher among the younger age groups, however; inevitably it will rise as these generations age. The figures show that a substantial proportion of older people is able to engage in a range of social, cultural and civic activities. It is up to organizations and policy makers to ensure that continued participation is facilitated and encouraged as people face more practical barriers to taking part in activities outside the home as they age. Engaging in a range of social activities, and the sense of inclusion and self-esteem this can offer, are important elements in improving older people's

Table 11.2 Civic participation, by gender

	Men	Women
Voted in the last election	83.9	81.5
Reads a daily newspaper	71.7	67.9
Has a hobby/pastime	78.9	76.9
Taken a holiday in UK in last 12 months	57.5	57.9
Gone on day trip in last 12 months	68.2	69.6
Use the Internet/email	36.3	25.7
Owns a mobile phone	60.1	55.0

Source: Marmot et al. (2003), Table 5A.21.

quality of life (Bowling *et al.* 2003). This is particularly true for people from minority ethnic communities (Nazroo 2002).

Loneliness and social isolation

Reduced social contact, being alone, isolation and feelings of loneliness are often associated with reduced quality in older people's lives (Victor *et al.* 2003). Increasing numbers of older people, especially older women, now live alone, as one partner outlives the other. Living alone, of course, is not synonymous with being lonely, although emerging evidence indicates that there is a clear association (Victor *et al.* 2000). However, feelings of loneliness can be experienced also by those living within larger households (Tunstall 1957), such as when a parent moves in with an adult child's family and lives in 'their' home or when an older person moves into residential care, where any surviving social networks may be disrupted or terminated.

Older people over the age of 65 in Britain and in some parts of Europe have consistently been found to report lower rates of loneliness than younger people (Walker and Maltby 1997; Victor *et al.* 2003). Self-reported measures used in early research into loneliness among older people in Britain revealed 7 per cent who said they were very lonely and 9 per cent who said they were often lonely (Sheldon 1948), however, self-reported rates of loneliness can under-represent the true extent of the problem because of the social stigma attached to it (Victor *et al.* 2000). Peer group studies of loneliness have dominated the research literature, especially for older people and later life. These seek to examine and measure the prevalence and distribution of loneliness amongst older people and to identify vulnerable groups from this. Victor and her colleagues (2003) argue that this is too static a measure and a more valid approach is to compare individuals' experience of loneliness in the present with their past experiences.

Recent research for the GO programme (Victor *et al.* 2003) used both self-reported measures of loneliness and indicators of participation and social contacts to examine the extent of the problem of loneliness, social isolation and living alone in later life. The research found that, overall, only a small minority of older people are lonely (7 per cent) or isolated (11–17 per cent) and that this has shown little change in the past 50 years. Any under-reporting of the problem was balanced against the high levels of contact with family, friends and neighbours, which most people had. The research identified vary-ing types and pathways into loneliness and isolation in later life and concluded that they must be understood if these problems are to be tackled effectively. The data from the study identified two distinct groups: those for whom loneliness is a continuation of previous experiences and those for whom it is a new experience.

A number of factors, including demographic variables as well as health, material and social resources, are implicated in the loneliness or isolation reported by older people. Vulnerability to loneliness is associated with poor mental health, poorer physical health, changes in perceived loneliness compared with the previous decade, and time spent alone. Advanced age and postbasic education appear to offer some protection against feelings of loneliness.

The role of services

Good community care services are important for older people to be able to live independently in their own homes and prevent deterioration in their QoL (Walker 1982; Walker and Warren 1996). Primary healthcare and social services inputs are equally important. In recent years social services depart-ments have faced reduced budgets and increasing demand for home-care services, resulting in the targeting of services on people with greatest need. This trend has also been encouraged by government policy. An emphasis on meeting high-level need has allowed prevention and rehabilitation work to suffer (Tanner 2001). However, older people value the input of low-intensity support services that may enable them to live independently for longer, an option that benefits health and social services as well as the older people. The Department of Health (1998) has formally recognized the need for more preventive service intervention, but such activities remain largely underdeveloped and uncoordinated (Tanner 2001).

As well as avoiding or delaying the admission into institutional care, preventive work with older people can also promote QoL by facilitating community engagement and social participation. This, together with the maintenance of a degree of independence, autonomy and reciprocity, contributes to a positive sense of identity and self-esteem among older people. Treating older people with respect and dignity, and without condescension, has been shown to be an inexpensive way to boost their QoL (George 1998). The concentration of services on very high risk groups, as well as virtually eliminating preventive work, has also encouraged practice that may undermine older people with urgent but nevertheless lower-level needs.

In 1997, the Department of Health funded a project, Shaping our Lives, as part of the Community Care Development Programme. Participants in the National User Group issued a Group Statement identifying equality, independence and empowerment as priorities in the provision of services. Being independent and empowered requires control and choice over one's lifestyle and particularly in the provision of support services (Walker and Warren 1996). Older people want to be able to have control over their lives and be responsible for how their days are organized but they do not necessarily see services as contributing to their QoL (Bowling 2003).

In their review of services, Qureshi and Henwood (2000) argue that the following proposals would have the greatest potential to contribute to older people's QoL:

- Better mobility inside and outside the home; achieved with adaptations to buildings, equipment, alternative housing, physiotherapy, mobility training for the visually impaired, and accessible transport.
- Reduction or management of symptoms of ill health such as lack of sleep, pain or incontinence.
- Better communications – to be achieved by the use of interpreters, audio tapes or Braille, hearing aids, speech therapy, teaching staff to use sign language, and reading letters out loud for blind older people.
- Regaining confidence and skills after trauma; regaining capability to look after oneself through training, counselling, physiotherapy and rehabilitation services.

♦ Higher benefit income to increase people's control over their capability to make choices and have control in their lives.

Older people have clear opinions on what kind of domiciliary services they need and how they should be delivered to promote QoL (Raynes *et al.* 2001). On the one hand, they want help with very small simple tasks around the home, such as replacing light bulbs, but they also want rather more fundamental changes at the organizational level, including:

♦ Continuity among carers and other services coming into the home to enable them to establish a relationship with service providers. This would give the older person more confidence in the service being provided and ensure that the service provider understands the needs, and preferences, of the older person. Constant changes of carer leave people feeling insecure and vulnerable as strangers constantly come into their home to undertake often very personal care tasks.

♦ Greater flexibility in service provision to adapt to changing needs and circumstances.

♦ Training for care staff, which includes listening to the older person whom they are supporting.

♦ Adaptations to houses and aids to help promote independence.

♦ Provision of transport services to facilitate outside contact with friends and relatives and to attend social clubs and other social events.

♦ Better healthcare services.

♦ Older people under 80 want more opportunities for social contact through the provision of places to meet people.

♦ The encouragement of 'good neighbours' by services.

♦ Older people from ethnic minority groups want services to respond to their cultural needs by promoting culturally specific activities, providing appropriate foods and making information available in minority languages.

♦ Regular meetings between the service user and the service care manager to monitor the quality of the home-care service provided, as well as three meetings per year in each of the areas, attended by service purchasers, providers, elected members and older people to hear the views of older people about service provision and their suggestions for improvements.

Life satisfaction and subjective wellbeing

Although the observation of a gap between the 'objective' living conditions of many older people and their frequently more optimistic subjective judgements is a longstanding issue in UK social gerontology (Townsend 1959, 1979; Walker 1980, 1990) there has been very little research into the self-reported life satisfaction of older people. Public-opinion style data suggest strong to slight satisfaction among just over half of older people in UK, close to the EU average (Midwinter 1991; Walker 1993) but detailed investigations have been undertaken only very recently.

What evidence there is suggests that attitudes towards QoL among older people are not very different to those of middle age, although there is some tendency for younger people to rate their QoL higher than other age groups, as Table 11.3 shows.

There are significant differences between older and younger people in terms of what they regard as important determinants of QoL (Bowling 1995, 1996). The population as a whole most frequently identifies relationships with family, friends and other people (53 per cent), followed closely by finances, standard of living and housing (48 per cent) and then own health (39 per cent), other people's health (32 per cent), ability to work/work satisfaction (26 per cent) and social life (17 per cent) (Bowling and Windsor 2001: 64). People aged 75 and over are more likely than younger respondents to prioritize their own health and the ability to

Table 11.3 Self-rated quality of life of different age groups (percentages)

Age groups	As good as can be	Very good	Good	Alright	Bad/very bad/as bad as can be	Total
16–24	14	36	37	11	2	100
25–34	17	27	34	19	3	100
35–44	17	30	30	21	2	100
45–54	16	34	29	17	4	100
55–64	20	27	33	18	2	100
65–74	22	30	28	16	4	100
75+	25	29	21	21	4	100

Source: Bowling and Windsor (2001) p. 65.

get out and about and are less likely to identify relationships with family and other relatives, finances and (not surprisingly) employment (Bowling 1996).

Further research has investigated the subjective opinions of older people about what constitutes 'good' and 'bad' quality in their lives (Bowling *et al.* 2002). The main items listed as maximizing QoL, as discussed in Chapter 6, were: having good health, retaining independence, psychological wellbeing and (positive) outlook, good relationships and contact with other people, adequate financial circumstances, home and neighbourhood characteristics and facilities, and social roles and activities.

Inequalities in quality of life

There are three well-documented structural inequalities in old age based on age, disability and gender. Evidence of a fourth, ethnicity, has emerged recently. Inequalities that can found during people's working lives generally persist into older age, and indeed can be exacerbated (Bardasi and Jenkins 2002). In Chapter 6, we considered the extent to which women are disadvantaged after retirement because of their work life histories of lower incomes and fewer working years and, therefore, inferior pensions. Inequalities in income often widen in old age as the value of pensions falls against the rising incomes of those still in work and those recently retired. Similarly, the lower average incomes of different ethnic minority communities persist into older age. Thus, Nazroo *et al.*'s (2003) GO research showed that, among people over the age of 50, people from the Pakistani ethnic minority group were twice (77 per cent) as likely to have incomes in the bottom third of (equivalized) income as the white population (36 per cent). Also 54 and 55 per cent of older people from Caribbean and Indian ethnic minority groups had incomes in the bottom third of the income distribution.

Nazroo *et al.*'s (2003) research also revealed extensive differences across ethnic groups in most influences on quality of life. Factors that the researchers regarded as typically associated with inequality – such as income and wealth, housing conditions and the physical environment – revealed a 'familiar pattern of inequality'. The white group had the highest scores, followed by the Indian and Caribbean groups, with the Pakistani group some way behind them. However, for those influences concerned with less formal elements of the community – social support and perceptions of local amenities – the differences were reversed, with older Pakistani people scoring higher than other groups. There was only slight variation in relation to crime.

Analysis of the quality of ELSA respondents' social ties revealed consistent gender differences and, to a lesser extent, differences by age and occupational status (Marmot *et al.* 2003: 313). Men across the age groups reported feeling closer to, and receiving more positive support from, their spouse or partner than did the women. Women reported more positive support from children, other relatives and friends than the men did, though positive support from friends fell as they got older. Negative support from all relationships – with spouse, children, other family members and friends, fell with increasing age, suggesting that people tend to view their relationships more positively as they get older or that there is a real improvement in how members of social networks relate to older people as they age.

Health

Inequalities in health are now recognized as being deeply entrenched in the UK. Data collected for ELSA (Marmot *et al.* 2003) reveal that age trends for certain occupational class groups imply that people in some occupational classes may experience long-standing poor health a decade or two earlier than those in more advantaged occupational classes. Men in routine and manual occupations are twice as likely to have poorer health than those in the professional and man-agerial classes between the ages of 50 and 59; the gap falls slightly between the ages of 60 to 74 and disappears over the age of 75. A similar pattern can be seen for women, though to a lesser degree. Occupational class differences in age trends were also found in heart disease, diagnosed hypertension (for men), diabetes, arthritis and respiratory illness (for men only). The authors argue that it is not possible to identify the underlying reasons for these socio-economic differences in age trends, although possible explanations could be an early ageing effect, selective survival (people in routine and manual occupations are more likely to die younger) or to a reduction in socio-economic influences on health at older ages (Marmot *et al.* 2003: 226). ELSA is to explore these important questions in future waves of the study.

Age trends in health-related behaviours, to some extent, mirrored the patterns shown for illness. Thus, men and women in routine and manual occupational classes were more likely to show sedentary behaviour (moderate or no vigorous activity) than those in professional and managerial groups. Older people up to the age of 80 in routine and manual occupations were approximately twice as likely to smoke as those in professional and managerial groups. After 80 this disparity levelled out. Men and women in manual house-holds were much more likely than their professional counterparts to abstain from drinking alcohol or to drink on special occasions only, whereas men and women in professional households were much more likely to drink moderately, in line with the pattern that is now thought to be protective against chronic illness (Marmot *et al.* 2003: 228).

Participation

The ELSA study explored participation in a number of cultural activities, such as going to the cinema, eating out, going to museums or art galleries, and going to the theatre or opera. The results show considerable disparities for going to the cinema, museum or art gallery and visiting the theatre or opera between the youngest and oldest age groups. Roughly twice as many in the youngest age group participate in such activities compared with those in the oldest age group. Poor health again was a factor in reducing participation at all age levels. The ELSA report (Marmot *et al.* 2003: 174) notes:

> clear occupational group differences in the rates of participation in cultural activities amongst the older population. In all age groups and for both sexes, there is a (sic) occupation class gradient in reporting going to the cinema, eating out of the house, visiting a museum or art gallery and going to the theatre or opera. The rate of going to the theatre or opera is over twice as great amongst men in the managerial and professional class . . . as amongst men from the routine and manual class.

This disparity is not surprising given the nature of the 'cultural activities' chosen. Participation by working-class people in such activities is no doubt lower across the lifespan. This is supported by the fact that fewer people in the routine and manual occupation classes reported that they engaged in these activities less than they wanted than respondents in either the intermediate or managerial and professional occupational classes. Except for state of health, the study did not explore the reasons why people were not able to participate in such activities as often as they wanted. Obvious reasons might be cost, reluctance to go out at night, difficulty in getting to places or getting access into theatres, or sensory impairment inhibiting enjoyment of a performance.

Future research priorities

As noted in Chapter 6, until recently UK research on QoL in old age was dominated by health-related definitions and investigations. This situation began to change in the late 1990s and there has been a substantial focus on this topic in recent years. A major reason for this interest stems from the government's

EQUAL programme launched in 1996. This was a virtual research programme spanning all of the UK's research councils and was focused on extending quality life. This led to specific research initiatives in all scientific disciplines, including the social sciences. The ESRC's GO Programme began in 1999 and ended in 2004. It comprised 24 individual projects spanning all of the key areas of QoL research:

◆ defining and measuring QoL;

◆ inequalities in QoL;

◆ technology and the built environment;

◆ health and productive ageing;

◆ family and support networks;

◆ participation and activity.

The programme has made a major contribution to the UK's portfolio of research on QoL in old age. Particularly important advances have been made in the definition and measurement of QoL, understanding QoL from the perspectives of gender and race, the roles of family and neighbourhood and the participation of older people. Despite this major boost to social science research on QoL in old age, and parallel research in the engineering and physical sciences disciplines, there are still important gaps in knowledge. Although there is no mechanism in the UK to set research priorities, the following areas require further investigation:

◆ the main dimensions of QoL and variations by age, gender and race;

◆ the roles and potential of ICT, housing and transport in determining QoL in old age (this dimension was under represented in the GO programme);

◆ how older people use their time;

◆ the role of employment in QoL among older workers;

◆ the changing life course and diversity in ageing;

◆ the relationship between locality and place and QoL;

◆ globalization, politics and ageing;

◆ saving and spending patterns in later life.

In addition there is a need in the UK to raise the scientific capacity to work with large data bases and to research numerically small populations of older people, such as those in advanced old age and in ethnic minority groups. There is also a need for more interdisciplinary collaboration in this field. The New Dynamics of Ageing Programme, sponsored by four UK research councils and covering all relevant scientific disciplines, which commenced in 2004, is aimed at filling a large proportion of these knowledge gaps and, in particular, at promoting interdisciplinary research.

Conclusion

This very brief review has emphasized the continuing high importance of family and wider social relationships in providing quality to older people's lives. While the pattern and nature of these relationships are changing, for example with regard to grandparenthood, they remain highly valued. Participation is relatively high among older people in the UK but differs according to gender, age, social class and disability. Minority ethnic groups value community (and family) participation more highly than their white counterparts. Services represent an important source of support but older people do not explicitly associate them with their QoL. There is a need to refocus social services on preventative support. Although recent research has shed a powerful light on the determinants of QoL in old age there are still aspects requiring further exploration, datasets to be exploited more fully and, especially, a need for interdisciplinary research.

References

Abele, A. and Becker, P. (eds) (1991) *Wohlbefinden: Theorie, Empirie, Diagnostik.* Munich: Juventa.

Abraham, E. (1993) *Arbeitstätigkeit, Lebenslauf und Pensionierung.* Münster: Waxmann.

Adler, G., Tremmel, S., Brassen, S., Scheib, A. (2000) Soziale Situation und Lebenszufriedenheit im Alter, *Zeitschrift für Gerontologie und Geriatrie,* 33(3): 210–16.

AGAST, Arbeitsgruppe Geriatrisches Assessment (1995) *Geriatrisches Basisassessment.* Munich: Handlungsanleitungen für die Praxis.

Allegato al Piano Sanitario Nazionale 1998–2000 (2000) Progetto Obiettivo Anziani. Unpublished manuscript, Ministero della Sanità, Rome.

Ancitel (2001) *Scenari di sviluppo per i servizi sociali e gli enti locali.* www.auser.it/STAMPA/AGENZIA/anno_4_numero_3_.htm.

Anderson, D.N. (2001) Treating depression in old age: the reasons to be positive, *Age and Ageing,* 30: 13–17.

Andersson, L. (1988) Elderly People in Nordic Time-Use Studies, in K. Altergott (ed.) *Daily Life in Later Life.* Newbury Park, CA: Sage Publications.

Andersson, L. (1993) *Äldre i Sverige och Europa,* Ädelutvärderingen, 93: 4, Stockholm: Socialstyrelsen (National Board of Health and Welfare).

Andersson, L. (1999) Social Isolation. Issue Report. Project Mégapoles – A public health network for capital cities/regions: Stockholm: Stockholm Gerontology Research Centre.

Andersson, L. (2002) Ålderism – några infallsvinklar in *Attåldras,* Bilagedel A till discussions betänkande "Riv ålderstrappan! Livslopp i forändring" (Sou 2002: 29). Stockholm: Fritzes.

Andersson, L. and Sundström, G. (1996) Social Networks of Elderly People in Sweden, in H. Litwin (ed.), *The Social Networks of Older People,* a cross-national analysis. Westport, CT: Praeger Publishing.

Antonucci, T.C., Sherman, A.M. and Akiyama, H. (1996) Social networks, support and integration, in J.E. Birren, *Encyclopedia of Gerontology*, 2. San Diego: Academic Press.

Arber, S. and Cooper, H. (1999) Gender differences in health in later life: the new paradox? *Social Science and Medicine*, 48, 61–76.

Askham, J., Nelson, H., Tinker, A. and Hancock, R. (1999) Older owner-occupiers' perceptions of home-ownership, *Joseph Rowntree Foundation Findings*. York: Joseph Rowntree Foundation.

Aureli, E. and Baldazzi, B. (1999) Soddisfazione e stili della vita anziana in Italia, in E. Aureli, F. Buratto, L. Carli Sardi, A. Franci, A. Ponti Sgargi and S. Schifini D'Andrea (eds) *Contesti di qualità di vita. Problemi e misure*. Milano: Franco Angeli.

Aust, B. (1994) *Zufriedene Patienten?* Berlin: WZB.

Avioli, P.S. (1989) The social support functions of siblings in later life: a theoretical model, *American Behavioral Scientist*, 33(1): 45–57.

Baldock, J. and Hadlow, J. (2002) *Housebound Older People: the Links between Identity, Self-esteem and the Use of Care Services*. Sheffield: Growing Older Programme, University of Sheffield.

Baltes, M.M. (1995) Verlust der Selbständigkeit im Alter, *Psychologische Rundschau*, 46: 159–70.

Baltes, P.B. and Baltes, M.M. (1990) Psychological perspectives on successful aging, in P.B. Baltes and M.M. Baltes (eds) *Successful Aging*. New York: Cambridge University Press.

Baltes, P.B. and Baltes, M.M. (1992) Gerontologie: Begriff, Herausforderung und Brennpunkte, in P.B. Baltes and J. Mittelstrass (eds) *Zukunft des Alterns und Gesellschaftliche Entwicklung*. Berlin: De Gruyter.

Baltes, M.M., Horgas, A.L., Klingenspor, B., Freund, A.M. and Carstensen, L.L. (1996a) Geschlechtsunterschiede in der Berliner Altersstudie, in K.-U. Mayer and P.B. Baltes (eds) *Die Berliner Altersstudie*. Berlin: Akademie-Verlag.

Baltes, M.M., Lang, F.R. and Wilms, H.-U. (1998) Selektive Optimierung mit Kompensation, in A. Kruse (ed.) *Psychosoziale Gerontologie. Band 1: Grundlagen*. Göttingen: Hogrefe.

Baltes, M.M., Maas, I., Wilms, H.-U. and Borchelt, M. (1996b) Alltagskompetenz im Alter, in K.U. Mayer and P.B. Baltes (eds) *Die Berliner Altersstudie*. Berlin:Akademie-Verlag.

Baltes, M.M. and Montada, L. (eds) (1996) *Produktives Leben im Alter*. Frankfurt am Main: Campus.

Baltes, M.M., Neumann, E.M. and Zank, S. (1994) Maintenance and rehabilitation of independence in old age, *Psychology and Aging*, 9: 179–88.

Baltes, M.M., Wahl, H.-W. and Reichert, M. (1991) Successful aging in long term care institutions, *Annual Review of Gerontology and Geriatrics*, 11: 311–37.

Baltes, P.B. (ed.) (1993) *Successful Aging: Perspectives from the Behavioural Sciences*. Cambridge: Cambridge University Press.

Banca d'Italia (2000) I bilanci delle famiglie italiane nell'anno 1998, *Supplementi al Bollettino Statistico*, Anno X (22).

Banfield, E.C. (1976) *Le basi morali di una società arretrata*. Bologna: Il Mulino.

Bardasi, E. and Jenkins, S. (2002) *Income in Later Life*. Bristol: Policy Press.

Beck, W., Van der Maesen, L. and Walker, A. (1997) (eds) *The Social Quality of Europe*. The Hague: Kluwer International.

Beck, W., Van der Maesen, L., Thomése, F. and Walker, A. (2001) (eds) *Social Quality: a Vision for Europe*. The Hague: Kluwer International.

Becker, P. (1982) *Psychologie der seelischen Gesundheit, Band 1: Theorien, Modelle, Diagnostik*. Göttingen: Hogrefe.

Becker, P. (1991) Theoretische Grundlagen, in A. Abele and P. Becker (eds) *Wohlbefinden: Theorie, Empirie, Diagnostik*. Munich: Juventa.

Becker, S., Lademann, J., Müller, K. and Thielborn, U. (1998) *Das Pflegegeschehen in der ambulanten Versangung aus Patientensicht*, Hochschulreform Pflege, 2(2): 15–17.

Beekman, A.T.F, Bremmer, M.A. and Deeg, D.J.H. (1998) Anxiety disorders in later life, *International Journal of Geriatric Psychiatry*, 13: 717–26.

Bengtson, V.L., Rosenthal, C. and Burton L. (1996) Paradoxes of family and aging, in R.H. Binstock and L.K. George (eds) *Handbook of Aging and the Social Sciences*, San Diego: Academic Press.

Berger-Schmitt, R. and Jankowitsch, B. (1999) *Systems of Social Indicators and Social Reporting: The State of the Art*. Mannheim: ZUMA.

Bernard, M. and Phillips, J. (2000) The challenge of ageing in tomorrow's Britain, *Ageing and Society*, 20: 33–54.

Bickel, H. (1995) Demenzkranke in Alten- und Pflegeheimen, in Friedrich-Ebert-Stiftung (ed.) *Medizinische und gesellschaftliche Herausforderungen: Alzheimer Krankheit*. Bonn: Friedrich-Ebert-Stiftung: 49–68.

Blinkert, B. and Klie, T. (1999) Pflege im sozialen Wandel. Eine Untersuchung über die Situation von häuslich versorgten Pflegebedürftigen nach Einführung der Pflegerversicherung. Hannover: Vincentz.

BMFSFJ (ed.) (1998) *Zweiter Bericht zur Lage der älteren Generation in der Bundesrepublik Deutschland*: *Wohnen im Alter*. Bonn: Deutscher Bundestag.

BMFSFJ (ed.) (2001a) *Dritter Bericht zur Lage der älteren Generation in der Bundesrepublik Deutschland. Alter und Gesellschaft*. Bonn: Deutscher Bundestag.

BMFSFJ (ed.) (2001b) *The Ageing of Society as a Global Challenge – German Impulses*. Berlin: Deutscher Bundestag.

BMFSFJ (ed.) (2002a) Vierter Bericht zur Lage der älteren Generation in der Bundesrepublik Deutschland: Risiken, Lebensqualität und Versorgung Hochaltriger – unter besonderer Berücksichtigung dementieller Erkrankungen. Berlin: Deutscher Bundestag.

BMFSFJ (ed.) (2002b) Modellprogramm 'Selbstbestimmt Wohnen im Alter' – drei Jahre Bundesmodellprogramm, *Newsletter* 12: 1–6.

Bogaerts, K. (2002) *Kwaliteit van leven van ouderen; een onderzoek naar definiëring en meetbaarheid*, Amsterdam: Vrije Universiteit (MA thesis).

Bond, J. (1999) Quality of life for people with dementia: approaches to the challenge of measurement, *Ageing and Society*, 19: 561–79.

Borchelt, M., Gilberg, R., Horgas, A.L. and Geiselmann, B. (1996) Zur Bedeutung von Krankheit und Behinderung im Alter, in K.U. Mayer and P.B. Baltes (eds) *Die Berliner Altersstudie*. Berlin: Akademie-Verlag.

Bowling, A. (1992) *Measuring Health*, Buckingham: Open University Press.

Bowling, A. (1995) What things are important in people's lives? A survey of the public's judgements to inform scales of health related quality of life, *Social Science and Medicine*, 41(10): 1447–62.

Bowling, A. (1996) The most important things in life, *International Journal of Health Sciences*, 6: 169–75.

Bowling, A. (2003) A taxonomy and overview of quality of life, in J. Brown, A. Bowling and T. Flynn (eds) Models of quality of life: a taxonomy and systematic review of the literature. Mimeo.

Bowling, A., Gabriel, Z., Banister, D. and Sutton, S. (2002) *Adding Quality to Quantity: Older People's Views on their Quality of Life and its Enhancement.* Sheffield: Growing Older Programme, University of Sheffield.

Bowling, A and Windsor, J. (2001) Towards the good life: a population survey of dimensions of quality of life, *Journal of Happiness Studies,* 2: 55–81.

Brandtstädter, J. and Greve, W. (1992) Das Selbst im Alter, *Zeitschrift für Entwicklungspsychologie und Pädagogische Psychologie,* 24(4): 1–20.

Brown, J., Bowling, A. and Flynn, T. (2003) Models of quality of life: a taxonomy and systematic review of the literature. Mimeo.

Buchmüller, R., Dobler, S., Kiefer, T., Margulies, F., Mayring, P., Melching, M. and Schneider, H.-D. (1996) *Vor dem Ruhestand. Eine psychologische Untersuchung zum Erleben der Zeit vor der Pensionierung.* Bern: Huber.

Buijssen, H. and Polspoel (1999) Rouw, in H. Buijssen (ed.), *Psychologische hulpverlening aan ouderen.* Baarn: HB Uitgevers.

Bulmahn, T. (1996) Determinanten des subjektiven Wohlbefindens, in W. Zapf and R. Habich (eds) *Wohlfahrtsentwicklung im vereinten Deutschland.* Berlin: Edition Sigma.

Burholt, V. and Wenger, C. (1998) Differences over time in older people's relationships with children and siblings, *Ageing and Society,* 18: 537–63.

Burholt, V., Wenger G.C., Lamura, G., Paulsson, C., Van der Meer, M., Ferring, D. and Glück, J. (2003) *European Study of Adult Wellbeing: Social Support Resources Comparative Report.* Report to European Commission, Centre for Social Policy Research and Development, University of Wales, Bangor.

Bytheway, B. (1987) Redundancy and the older worker, in R.M. Lee (ed.), *Redundancy, Layoffs and Plant Closures.* Beckenham: Croom Helm.

Campbell, A. (1983) *The Sense of Wellbeing in America.* New York: McGraw-Hill.

Campbell, N. (1999) *The Decline of Employment Among Older People in Britain.* London: LSE, Centre for Analysis of Social Exclusion.

Carbonin, P., Manto, A., Pahor, M., Pedone, C. and Carosella, L. e i ricercatori del GIFA (1997) Il ricorso ai servizi sanitari, in *La salute degli anziani in Italia, collana Monografie,* 7, Rome: IRP: 91–108.

Cariani, G., Gamberoni, M. and Hanau, C. (1997) L'influenza dell'età sul ricorso ai servizi sanitari, in *La salute degli anziani in Italia. collana Monografie,* 7, Rome: IRP: 111–28.

Caritas and Migrantes (2003) *Dossier Statistico Immigrazione 2003*. Rome: Anterem.

Carley, M. (1981) *Social Measurement and Social Indicators*, London: Allen & Unwin.

Carvel, J. (2001) Crime is the key issue for older people, says poll, *The Guardian*, 23 September 2001.

Casey, B. and Laczko, F. (1989) Early retired or long-term unemployed? The situation of non-working men aged 55–64 from 1976 to 1986, *Work Employment and Society*, 1(4): 509–26.

Cataldi, L. (1996) L'assistenza agli anziani nella regione Emilia Romagna, in *Politiche familiari welfare e sviluppo sostenibile*. Rome: IRP-CNR.

Cataldi, V. and Ricci, S. (2000) L'andamento dei tassi di attività e di disoccupazione degli ultracinquantenni in Europa, in G. Geroldi (ed.) *Lavorare da anziani e da pensionati*. Milano: Franco Angeli.

CBS (2000) Allochtonen, 1 januari 2000, *Maandstatistiek van de bevolking*, 9: 22–86.

CBS (2000) Bevolking van Nederland naar burgerlijke staat, geslacht en leeftijd, *Maandstatistiek van de bevolking*, 8: 19–22.

CBS (2001) *Kerngegevens leefsituatie 2000*, Voorburg: Centraal Bureau voor de Statistiek.

CENSIS (2001) *Primo rapporto annuale sulla comunicazione in Italia*. Rome. See www. gandalf.it/dati/censis.htm.

CENSIS/Forum per la ricerca biomedica (2002) *Le garanzia per la salute tra globalizzazione e localismo*. Rome. (See also www.ministerosalute.it/dettaglio/pdPrimoPiano.jsp?id=16&sub=0&lang=it.)

Cesa Bianchi M. and Cristini, C.A. (1998) Qualità della vita, in G. Cesa Bianchi and T. Vecchi (eds) *Elementi di psico-gerontologia*. Milano: Franco Angeli.

Cicirelli, V.G. (1991) The longest bond: the sibling life cycle in L. L'Abate (ed.) *Handbook of Developmental Family Psychology and Psychopathology*. New York: John Wiley and Sons.

Clarke, L. and Roberts, C. (2003) *Grandparenthood: Its Meaning and Its Contribution to Older People's Lives*, Sheffield: Growing Older Programme, University of Sheffield.

Clemens, W. (1995) *Zur Lebenslage erwerbstätiger Frauen zwischen Arbeit und Rente*. Freie Universität Berlin: Habilitationsschrift.

Closs, C., and Kempe, P. (1986) Eine differenzierende Betrachtung und Validierung des Konstrukts Lebenszufriedenheit, *Zeitschrift für Gerontologie*, 19: 47–55.

Clough, R. (1996) Homes for heroines and heroes? Hotels for pensioners? Housing and care for older people. Inaugural lecture, Lancaster University.

CNEL – Consiglio Nazionale dell'Economia e del Lavoro (2000) *Agenda degli Italiani*. Rome: CNEL.

Connidis, I.A. (1989) Siblings as friends in later life, *American Behavioral Scientist*, 33(1): 81–93.

Cuijpers, P. (1999) Het actief aanbieden van behandeling aan depressieve ouderen, *Psychopraxis*, 1: 76–8.

Dannenbeck, C. (1995) Im Alter einsam? Zur Strukturveränderung sozialer Beziehungen im Alter, in H. Bertram (ed.) *Das Individuum und seine Familie*. Opladen: Leske & Budrich.

De Beer, J., De Jong, A. and Visser, H. (1993) Nationale Huishoudprognose 1993 (National Household Forecast, 1993), *Maandstatistiek van de Bevolking*, 93(8): 13–23.

De Beurs, E., Beekman, A.T.F. and Deeg, D.J.H. (2000) Predictors of change in anxiety symptoms of older persons, *Psychological Medicine*, 30: 515–27.

De Jong Gierveld, J. (1999) Older adults between family solidarity and independence. Paper presented at the PAA, 1999, Annual Meeting, New York.

De Jong Gierveld, J. and Van Tilburg, T.G. (1995) Social relationships, integration and loneliness, in C.P.M. Knipscheer, J. de Jong Gierveld, T.G. van Tilburg and P.A. Dykstra, *Living Arrangements and Social Networks of Older Adults*. Amsterdam: VU University Press.

De Jong Gierveld, J. (1989) Personal relationships, social support, and loneliness, *Journal of Social and Personal Relationships*, 6: 197–221.

De Vincenti, C. (ed.) (2000) *Gli anziani in Europa*. IX Rapporto CER-SPI. Bari: Edizioni Laterza.

De Vincenti, C. and Minelli, R. (eds) (2001b) *Famiglia, assistenza, fisco*. XI Rapporto CER-SPI. Rome: Ediesse.

De Vincenti, C. and Rodano, G. (eds) (2001c) *Venti anni di transizione dell'economia italiana*. XII Rapporto CER-SPI. Rome: Ediesse.

Dean, M. (2003) *Growing Older in the 21st Century*. Swindon: ESRC.

Decreto del Ministero della Sanità del 14 dicembre 1994, Tariffe delle prestazioni di assistenza ospedaliera. Rome.

Deeg, D.J.H. and Westendorp-de Serière, M. (eds) (1994) *Autonomy and Wellbeing in the Aging Population I*. Amsterdam: VU University Press.

Deeg, D.J.H., Beekman, A.T.F., Kriegsman, D.M.W. and Westendorp-de Serière, M. (eds) (1998) *Autonomy and Wellbeing in the Aging Population II*. Amsterdam: VU University Press.

Deeg, D.J.H., Bosscher, R.J., Broese van Groenou, M.I. *et al.* (2000) *Ouder Warden in Nederland: Tien Jaar Longitudinal Aging Study Amsterdam (LASA)*. Amsterdam: Thela Thesis.

Dekker, P. and Van den Broek, A. (1998) Civil society in comparative perspective, *Voluntas: International Journal of Voluntary and Nonprofit Organizations*, 9(1): 11–38.

Delai, N. (1998) *Essere anziano oggi*. Rome: Editore Cinquanta & Più.

Delai, N. (1999) *Essere anziano oggi. Identità, consumi e valori dell'età matura*. Rome: Editore Cinquanta & Più.

Delai, N. (2000) *Essere anziano oggi*. Rome: Editore Cinquanta & Più.

Delai, N. (2001) E' ora di 'sdoganare' l'età matura, *Il Sole 24 Ore*, 2 December.

Delhey, J., Bhuk, P., Habich, R. and Zapf, W. (2001) *The Euromodule. A New Instrument for Comparative Welfare Research*. Berlin: WZB.

Delhey, J. and Böhnke, P. (1999) *Über die materielle zur inneren Einheit?* Berlin: WZB.

Department for Transport, Local Government and the Regions (2001) *Older People: Their Transport Needs and Requirements*. London: Department for Transport, Local Government and the Regions.

Department for Work and Pensions (2001) *Income-related Benefits: Estimates of Take-up 1999–2000*. London: DWP.

Department for Work and Pensions (2002) *Opportunity for All: Fourth Annual Report*, CM. 5598. London: The Stationery Office.

Department of Health (1998) *Our Healthier Nation*. London: The Stationery Office.

Department of the Environment, Transport and the Regions (2001) *Quality and Choice for Older People's Housing – A Strategic Framework*. http://www.housing.detr.gov.uk/information/hsc/olderpeople/11/htm.

Dietzel-Papakyriakou, M. (1998) Ältere Migranten, in Deutsches Rotes Kreuz Generalsekretariat (ed.) *Alt in der Fremde, fremd im Alter? Tagungsdokumentation*. Bonn: Eigenverlag: 9–25.

Dietzel-Papakyriakou, M. and Olbermann, E. (1996) Soziale Netzwerke älterer Migranten, *Zeitschrift für Gerontologie und Geriatrie*, 29(1): 34–41.

Dijk, L van, de Haan, J. and Rijken, S. (2000) *Digitalisering van de leefwereld; een onderzoek naar informatie*, Den Haag: Sociaal en Cultureel Planbureau.

Dinkel, R. (1999) Demographische Entwicklung und Gesundheitszustand, in H. Häfner (ed.) *Gesundheit – unser höchstes Gut?* Berlin: Akademie-Verlag.

Disney, R., Grundy, E. and Johnson, P. (1997) *The Dynamics of Retirement*. London: HMSO.

Dittmann-Kohli, F. (1995) *Das Persönliche Sinnsystem*. Göttingen: Hogrefe.

Draper, M.B.B.S. (1999) The diagnosis and treatment of depression in dementia, *Psychiatric Services*, 50: 1151–3.

Driest, P. and Weekers, S. (1998) *Persoonsgebonden budget*. Utrecht: NIZW.

Droogleever Fortuijn, J., Van der Meer, M., Sassenrath, S *et al.* (2003) *Comparative Report on Ageing Well and Life Activities*. Report to European Commission, Centre for Social Policy Research and Development, University of Wales, Bangor.

Ds (2002) Gyllene år med silverhår – för vissa eller för alla? Stockholm: Fritzes.

Dugan and Kivett (1994) The importance of emotional and social isolation to loneliness among very old rural adults, *Gerontologist*, 34(3): 340.

Dykstra P.A. and De Jong Gierveld, J. (1999) Differentiële kansen op eenzaamheid onder ouderen, *Tijdschrift voor Gerontologie en Geriatrie*, 30(5): 212–25.

Dykstra, P.A. (1995) Age differences in social participation, in C.P.M. Knipscheer, J. de Jong Gierveld, T.G. van Tilburg and P.A. Dykstra (eds) *Living Arrangements and Social Networks of Older Adults*. Amsterdam: VU University Press.

Dykstra, P.A. and Knipscheer, C.P.M. (1995) The availability and intergenerational structure of family relationships, in C.P.M. Knipscheer, J. de Jong Gierveld, T.G. van Tilburg and P.A. Dykstra, *Living Arrangements and Social Networks of Older Adults*. Amsterdam: VU University Press.

ERC-ECMT (2000) *Transport and Ageing of the Population*. Paris: OECD Publications Service.

Ernst, J. (1996) Vom Vorruhestand in den Ruhestand – Wandel und Stabilität der sozialen Lage ostdeutscher Frührentner, *Zeitschrift für Gerontologie und Geriatrie*, 29(5): 352–5.

ESIS-ISPO (2000) *Information Society Indicators in the Member States of the European Union*. Brussels.

ETAN (1998) *Ageing Population and Technology*. Brussels: European Commission.

EURISPES-SIP (1993) *Terzo Rapporto sulla condizione degli anziani in Italia*. Rome. (See also www.mix.it/Eurispes/EURISPES/168/default.htm.)

Eurobarometer (2003) *Standard Eurobarometer 59 – Spring 2003*. Brussels: EC.

Eurolink Age (2000) *Older People in the European Union: Facts and Figures*. London.

European Commission (2001) *The Social Situation in the European Union*. Luxembourg: Office for Official Publications of the European Communities.

European Commission (2003) *The Social Situation in the European Union*. Luxembourg: Office for Official Publications of the European Communities.

EUROSTAT (2000) *European Social Statistics – Demography*. Luxembourg: Office for Official Publications of the European Communities.

Evers, A. and Rauch, U. (1998) Pfleglichkeit und Nutzerorientierung. Bericht der wissenschaftlichen Begleitforschung des Modellprojekts 'Pflege im Vogelsbergkreis'. Lauterbach: Koordinierunsstelle für ambulante pflegendienste des Landratsamts des Vogelbergkreises.

Everwien, S. (1992) *Lebenszufriedenheit bei Frauen*. Münster: Waxmann.

Fachinger, U. (1998) *Die Verteilung der Vermögen privater Haushalte*. Bremen: Zentrum für Sozialpolitik, Universität Bremen.

Fachinger, U. (2001) Materielle Ressourcen älterer Menschen, in Deutsches Zentrum für Altersfragen (DZA) (ed.) *Erwerbsbiographien und materielle Lebenssituation im Alter*, Band 2. Opladen: Leske & Budrich.

Farrington, J.H. (ed.) (1999) *Rural Transport*, Aberdeen: Arkleton Centre for Rural Development Research.

Ferilli, A.M., Arsie, P., Baretter, A. *et al.* (2000) Trattamento psico-sociale del disturbo depressivo in anziani istituzionalizzati, *Giornale di Gerontologia*, 6: 357–8.

Fernández-Ballesteros, R., Zamarrón, M., and Ruíz, M. (2001) The contribution of socio-demographic and psychosocial factors to life satisfaction, *Ageing and Society*, 21(1): 25–44.

Ferring, D. and Filipp, S.-H. (1997a) Retrospektive Bewertungen des eigenen Lebens, *Zeitschrift für Entwicklungspsychologie und Pädagogische Psychologie*, 29(1): 83–95.

Ferring, D. and Filipp, S.-H. (1997b) Subjektives Wohlbefinden im Alter, *Psychologische Beiträge*, 39: 236–58.

Ferring, D. and Filipp, S.-H. (1999) Soziale Netze im Alter, *Zeitschrift für Entwicklungspsychologie und Pädagogische Psychologie*, 31: 127–37.

Ferring, D., Hallberg, I.R., Hoffman, M. *et al.* (2003) *Physical Health and Functional Status – European Study of Adult Wellbeing*. Report to European Commission, Centre for Social Policy Research and Development, University of Wales, Bangor.

Ferring, D., Wenger, G.C., Hoffmann, M. *et al.* (2003a) *Comparative Report on the European Model of Ageing Well*. Report to European Commission, Centre for Social Policy Research and Development, University of Wales, Bangor.

Filipp, S.H., Ferring, D., Mayer, A.K. and Schmidt, K. (1997) Selbstbewertungen und selektive Präferenz für temporale vs. soziale Vergleichsinformation bei alten und sehr alten Menschen, *Zeitschrift für Sozialpsychologie*, 28: 30–43.

Fillenbaum, G.G. (1988) *Multidimensional Functional Assessment of Older Adults*. Hillsdale: Lawrence Erlbaum Associates.

Flick, U. (ed.) (1998) *Wann fühlen wir uns gesund? Subjektive Vorstellungen von Gesundheit und Krankheit*. Weinheim: Juventa.

Fliege, H. and Filipp, S.-H. (2000) Subjektive Theorien zu Glück und Lebensqualität. Ergebnisse explorativer Interviews mit 65- bis 74 jährigen, *Zeitschrift für Gerontologie und Geriatrie*, 33(4): 307–13.

Florea, A. (1994) Vita familiare e relazionale, in *Ministero dell'Interno – ISTISS*. Rome: Ministero dell'Interno – Direzione Generale dei Servizi Civili.

Fokkema, C.M. and De Jong Gierveld, J. (1999) Beter een goede buur dan een verre vriend? *Demos*, 15(5).

Folkhälsorapport 2001 (2001) *Äldres hälsa och välbefinnande*. Stockholm: Stockholm Gerontology Research Center.

Forsell, Y. (2000a) Death wishes in the very elderly, *Acta Psychiatrica Scandinavica*, 102: 135–8.

Forsell, Y. (2000b) Predictors for depression, anxiety and psychotic symptoms in a very elderly population, *Soc Psychiatry Psychiatr Epidemiol*, 35: 259–63.

Forum degli Assessorati ai Servizi Sociali (1997) *Sintesi dei principali risultati del rapporto*. www.auser.it/Allegati/Genova/documenti.htm.

Foschi, F. and Barbini, N. (2000) Il lavoro e l'invecchiamento della popolazione nel nuovo millennio, *Difesa Sociale*, 3–4: 141–52.

Fowkes, A., Oxley, P. and Heiser, B. (1994) *Cross-sector Benefits of Accessible Public Transport* (report). Cranfield: Cranfield University, School of Management.

Franci, A. and Corsi, M. (1996) *La qualità soggettiva dell'assistenza residenziale agli anziani*. Padova: Edizioni Summa.

Frese, M. (1990) Arbeit und Emotion – ein Essay, in F. Frei and I. Udris (eds) *Das Bild der Arbeit*. Bern: Huber.

Freudenthal, A. (1999) *The Design of Home Appliances for Young and Old Consumers*. Delft: Technische Universiteit, Delft.

Freund, A. and Baltes, P. (1998) Selection, Optimisation and Compensation as Strategies of Life Management, *Psychology and Aging*, 13: 531–43.

Freund, A.M. (1995) *Die Selbstdefinition alter Menschen*. Berlin: Sigma.

Freund, A.M. and Smith, J. (1997) Die Selbstdefinition im hohen Alter, *Zeitschrift für Sozialpsychologie*, 28: 44–59.

Frey, L. (ed.) (1997) Formazione e benessere degli anziani in Italia, *Quaderni di Economia del Lavoro*, 60-numero monografico. Milano: Franco Angeli.

Frey, L. (1999) La solidarietà intergenerazionale, *OggiDomaniAnziani*, 2: 13–56.

Frey, L. (2000a) L'invecchiamento attivo in Europa, *Il benessere degli anziani* 4: 1–8.

Frey, L. (2000b) Il reddito degli anziani in Italia a fine anni '90, *Il benessere degli anziani*, 6: 1–8.

Frey, L. (2001a) Diritto all'istruzione/apprendimento e benessere delle persone avanti nell'età, *Il benessere degli anziani*, 3–4: 1–11.

Frey, L. (2001b) Assistenza domiciliare: tenere il passo con l'Europa, *Il benessere degli anziani*, 9: 1–8.

Frey, L. (2002) La povertà degli anziani in Italia, *Il benessere degli anziani*, 2: 1–8.

Frey, L. and Livraghi R. (1999) Famiglia e solidarietà tra le generazioni, in Federazione Nazionale Pensionati Cisl (ed.) *Anziani '98 – Tra uguaglianza e diversità*. Rome: Edizioni Lavoro.

Fuchs, R., Hahn, A. and Schwarzer, R. (1994) Effekte sportlicher Aktivität auf Selbstwirksamkeits-Erwartung und Gesundheit in einer stressreichen Lebenssituation, *Sportwissenschaft*, 24: 67–81.

Gabriel, Z. and Bowling, A. (2004) Quality of life in old age from the perspectives of older people, in A. Walker and C. Hagan Hennessy (eds) *Growing Older: Quality of Life in Old Age*. Maidenhead: Open University Press.

Geerlings, M.I. (2000) *Depression, memory complaints, education and Alzheimer's disease*. Amsterdam: Vrije Universiteit, faculteit geneeskunde (proefschift).

Genz, M. (1995) Veränderungen und Kontinuitäten der Lebenslage und des Gesundheitszustandes älterer Menschen zwischen 1989 und 1992, in H. Bertram, S. Hradil and G. Kleinhenz (eds) *Sozialer und demographischer Wandel in den neuen Bundesländern*. Berlin: Akademie Verlag.

Geroldi, G. (ed.) (2000) *Lavorare da anziani e da pensionati*. Milano: Franco Angeli.

Gilgen, R.U. and Garms-Homolóva, V. (1995) Resident Assessment Instrument (RAI), *Zeitschrift für Gerontologie und Geriatrie*, 2: 25–8.

Gilhooly, M., Hamilton, K., O'Neill, M., Gow, J., Webster, N. and Pike, F. (2003) *Transport and Ageing: Extending Quality of Life via Public and Private Transport*. Sheffield: Growing Older Programme, University of Sheffield.

Gilleard, C. and Higgs, P. (2001) *Cultures of Ageing*, Harlow: Prentice Hall.

Ginn, J. and Arber, S. (1995) Only connext: gender relations and ageing, in S. Arber and J. Ginn (eds) *Connecting Gender and Ageing: A Sociological Approach*, Buckingham: Open University Press.

Ginn, J. and Arber, S. (1996) Gender, age and attitudes to retirement in mid-life, *Ageing and Society*, 16: 27–55.

Ginn, J. and Arber, S. (1999) Changing patterns of pension inequality: the shift from state to private sources, *Ageing and Society*, 19: 319–42.

Glatzer, W. (1992) Lebensqualität und subjektives Wohlbefinden. Ergebnisse sozialwissenschaftlicher Untersuchungen, in A. Bellebaum (ed.) *Glück und Zufriedenheit*. Opladen: Westdeutscher Verlag.

Glatzer, W. (1998) Lebensstandard und Lebensqualität, in B. Schäfers and W. Zapf (eds) *Handwörterbuch zur Gesellschaft Deutschlands*. Opladen: Leske & Budrich.

Glatzer, W. and Allmendinger, J. (1999) *Deutschland im Wandel*. Opladen: Leske & Budrich.

Glatzer, W. and Volkert, M. (1980) Lebensbedingungen und Lebensqualität alter Menschen. *Zeitschrift für Gerontologie*, 13(3): 247–60.

Glatzer, W. and Zapf, W. (eds) (1984) *Lebensqualität in der Bundesrepublik*. Frankfurt am Main: Campus.

Golini, A. and Bruno, P. (1999) Tendenze demografiche, invecchiamento della popolazione e impatto sull'ambiente, in R. Colantonio, M. Lucchetti and A. Venturelli (eds) *Ambiente e invecchiamento*. Milano: Guerini Studio.

Golini, A. and Calvani, P. (1997) Un paese dalle politiche povere in le persone anziane. *Protagonisti a tutti gli effetti, Famiglia Oggi*, 12.

Goodman, A., Myck, M. and Shephard, A. (2003) *Sharing the Nation's Prosperity? Pensioner poverty in Britain*. London: Institute for Fiscal Studies.

Gori, C. (ed.) (2001a) *I servizi sociali in Europa*. Rome: Carocci Editore.

Gori, C. (ed.) (2001b) *Le politiche per gli anziani non autosufficienti*. Milano: Franco Angeli.

Gori, C. and Torri, R. (2001) Gli assegni di cura in Italia, in C. Ranci (ed.) *L'assistenza agli anziani in Italia e in Europa*. Milano: Franco Angeli.

Görres, S. (1999) *Qualitätssicherung in Pflege und Medizin. Bestandsaufnahme, Theorieansätze, Perspektiven*. Bern, Göttingen: Huber.

Grammarota, G. (1996) Le università della terza età: un'indagine Auser, in V. Gallina and M. Lichtner (eds) *L'educazione in età adulta*. Milano: Franco Angeli.

Griffiths, R. (1988) *Community Care: Agenda for Action*. London: HMSO.

Grillo, F. (2001) *Il ritorno della rete*. Rome: Fazi Editore.

Grundy, E. and Bowling, A. (1999) Enhancing the quality of extended life years. *Ageing and Mental Health*, 3(3): 199–212.

Gubrium, J. and Lynott, R. (1983) Rebuilding Life Satisfaction, *Human Organisation*, 42(1): 33–8.

Guillemard, A.-M. (1993) Travailleurs vieillessants et marché de travail en Europe, *Travail et Emploi*, 57: 60–79.

Gussekloo, J., De Craen, A.J.M. and Westendorp, R.G.J. (2000) Reden tot optimisme, *Medisch contact*, 13: 473–6.

Habich, R., Noll, H.-H. and Zapf, W. (1999) Subjektives Wohlbefinden in Ostdeutschland nähert sich westdeutschem Niveau, *Informationsdienst Soziale Indikatoren*, 22: 1–6.

Hagestad, G. (1985) Older women in inter-generational relations in M.R. Haung, A.B. Ford and M. Sheafer (eds) *The Physical and Mental Health of Aged Women*. New York: Springer.

Hancock, R. and Wright, F. (1999) Older couples and long-term care: the financial implications of one spouse entering private or voluntary residential or nursing home care, *Ageing and Society*, 19: 209–37.

Hanson, J. (2001) From 'special needs' to 'lifestyle choices': articulating the demand for 'third age' housing, in S. Peace and C. Holland (eds) *Inclusive Housing in an Ageing Society*. Southampton: Policy Press.

Hauser, R., Glatzer, W., Hradil, S., Kleinhenz, G., Olk, T. and Pankoke, E. (1996) *Ungleichheit und Sozialpolitik*. Opladen: Leske & Budrich.

Hautzinger, M. and Kleine, W. (1995) Sportliche Aktivität und psychisches Wohlbefinden, Zur Wirkung von Sport auf depressive Symptomatik, *Zeitschrift für Gesundheitspsychologie*, 3: 255–67.

Heinemann-Knoch, M., Korte, E., Schönberger, Ch. and Schwarz, B. (1999) *Möglichkeiten und Grenzen selbständigen Lebens und Arbeitens in stationären Einrichtungen*. Schriftenreihe des BFSFJ. Stuttgart: Kohlhammer.

Heinze, R.G., Eichener, V., Naegele, G., Bucksteeg, M. and Schauerte, M. (1997) *Neue Wohnung auch im Alter*. Darmstadt: Schader-Stiftung.

Helmchen, H., Baltes, H.H., Geiselmann, B. *et al.* (1996) Psychische Erkrankungen im Alter, in K.U. Mayer and P.B. Baltes (eds) *Die Berliner Altersstudie*. Berlin: Akademie-Verlag.

Help the Aged (2003) *Older People Count: The Help the Aged Income Index for Older People in England and Wales 2003*. London: Help the Aged.

Hendriks, G.J., Keijsers, G.P.J. and Hoogduin, C.A.L. (1999) Cognitieve gedragstherapie bij ouderen met angststoornissen, *Tijdschrift voor psychiatrie* 41(11): 677–81.

Henkens, C.J.M. (2001) Met pensioen en toch een baan? *Demos*, 18(1): 1–4.

Heyl, V., Oswald, F., Ziprich, D., Wetzler, R. and Wahl, H.-W. (1997) *Bedürfnisstrukturen älterer Menschen*. Heidelberg: DZFA.

Hillerås, P., Jorm, A., Herlitz, A. and Winblad, B. (1998) Negative and positive affect among the very old, *Research on Aging*, 20: 593–610.

Hillerås, P., Jorm, A., Herlitz, A. and Winblad, B. (1999) Activity patterns in very old people, *Age and Ageing*, 28: 147–52.

Hillerås, P., Jorm, A., Herlitz, A. and Winblad, B. (2001) Life satisfaction among the very old, *International Journal of Aging and Human Development*, 52: 71–90.

Hillerås, P., Pollitt, P., Medway, J. and Ericsson, K. (2000) Nonagenarians, *Ageing and Society*, 20: 673–97.

Hine, J., Sean, D., Scott, J., Binnie, D. and Sharp, J. (2000) Using Technology to overcome the Tyranny of Space: Information Provision and Wayfinding, *Urban Studies*, 37(10): 1757–70.

Hinrichs, W. (1997) *Wohnbedingungen und ihre subjektive Wahrnehmung in Ostdeutschland 1990–1997*. Berlin: WZB.

Hinrichs, W. (1999) *Entwicklung der Wohnverhältnisse in Ost- und Westdeutschland in den neunziger Jahren*. Berlin: WZB.

House, J.S. and Kahn, R.L. (1985) Measures and concepts of social support, in S. Cohenand and S.L. Syme (eds) *Social Support and Health*. Orlando: Academic Press.

Hughes, B. (ed.) (1990) *Quality of Life, in Researching Social Gerontology*. London: Sage Publications.

Il Sole – 24 Ore del Lunedì (2003) *La qualità della vita nelle province italiane*. www.comune.bologna.it/iperbole/piancont/archivionov/tabelle_grafici/quali-tasole2003/classifica_finale.PDF.

Ipso Facto en SGBO (2001) *Een verstrekkende wet 3*. Den Haag: Ministerie van Sociale Zaken en Werkgelegenheid.

IRP-CNR (1997) La salute degli anziani in Italia, *Collana monografie* www.aging.cnr.it/indexgb.htm.

IRP-CNR/Palomba, R., Misiti, M. and Sabatino, D. (eds) (2001) *La vecchiaia può attendere*, *Demotrends*, 1 March.

ISTAT (1997) *Anziani in Italia*. Bologna: Il Mulino.

ISTAT (1999a) *Gli incidenti domestici. Serie 'Statistiche in breve'*. www.auser.it/Allegati/Genova/documenti.htm.

ISTAT (1999b) *European Community Household Panel (ECHP). Serie 'Statistiche in breve'*. Rome.

ISTAT (2000a) *I servizi pubblici e di pubblica utilità: utilizzo e soddisfazione*. Rome: Collana Informazioni.

ISTAT (2000b) *Le condizioni di salute degli italiani. Anno 1999. Serie 'Statistiche in breve'*. Rome.

ISTAT (2000c) *Cause di morte. Anno 1997. Serie 'Sanità e previdenza', Annuario n. 13*. Rome.

ISTAT (2001a) *Famiglie, abitazioni e sicurezza dei cittadini. Anno 2000*. Rome.

ISTAT (2001b) *Stili di vita e condizioni di salute. Anno 2000*. Rome: Collana Informazioni.

ISTAT (2001c) *Parentela e reti di solidarietà. Anno 1998*. Rome: Collana Informazioni.

ISTAT (2001d) *Cultura, socialità e tempo libero. Anno 2000*. Rome: Collana Informazioni.

ISTAT (2001e) *Rapporto sull'Italia 2001*. Bologna: Il Mulino.

ISTAT (2003) *Annuario Statistico Italiano*. Rome.

Jerrome, D. (1994) Time, change and continuity in family life, *Ageing and Society*, 14: 1–27.

Johansson, I. (1997) *Ålder och arbete*. Stockholm: Stockholms universitet, Pedagogiska institutionen.

Johansson, L. (2000) Social protection for dependency in old age in Sweden, in J. Pacolet and R. Bouten (eds) *Social Protection for Dependency in Old Age*. Leuven: Hoger Instituut voor de Arbeid.

Johnson, M. (1976) That was your life: a biographical approach to later life, in J.M.A. Munnichs and W.J.A. Van Den Heuvel (eds), *Dependency and Interdependency in Old Age*. The Hague: Martinus Nijhoff.

Johnson, T. (1995) Ageing well in contemporary society: introduction, *American Behavioural Scientist*, 39(2): 120–30.

Jones, G. (1987) Elderly People and Domestic Crime: Reflections on Ageism, Sexism and Victimology, *British Journal of Criminology*, 27(2): 191–201.

Jönson, H. (2001) *Det moderna åldrandet*. Lund Dissertations in Social Work 2. Lund: Lunds universitet, Socialhögskolan.

Jönson, H. and Magnusson, J.A. (2001) A new age of old age? *Journal of Aging Studies*, 15: 317–31.

Kerrison, S. and Pollock, A.M., (2001) Absent voices compromise the effectiveness of nursing home regulation: a critique of regulatory reform in the UK nursing home industry, *Health and Social Care in the Community*, 9(6): 490–4.

Kickbusch, I. (1999) Der Gesundheitsbegriff der Weltgesundheitsorganisation, in H. Häfner (ed.) *Gesundheit – unser höchstes Gut?* Berlin, Heidelberg: Springer.

Kingston, P., Bernard, M., Biggs, S., and Nettleton, H., (2001) Assessing the health impact of age-specific housing, *Health and Social Care in the Community* 9(4): 228–34.

Kinsella, K., Velkoff, V.A. and U.S. Census Bureau (2001) *An Ageing World: 2001*. Series P95/01–1. Washington DC: US Printing Office,

Klerk, M.M.Y. de, and Timmermans, J.M. (eds) (1999) *Rapportage ouderen 1998*. Den Haag: Sociaal en Cultureel Planbureau/Elsevier bedrijfsinformatie.

Kliegel, M., Rott, Ch., d'Heureuse, V., Becker, G. and Schönemann, P. (2001) Demenz im höchsten Alter ist keine Notwendigkeit. Ergebnisse der Heidelberger Hundertjährigen-Studie, *Zeitschrift für Gerontopsychologie und -psychiatrie*, 14(4): 169–80.

Knipscheer, C.P.M. (1996) Maatschappelijke participatie van ouderen, in K. Penninx. *Ongekend talent*. Utrecht: Nederlands Instituut voor Zorg en Welzijn.

Knipscheer, C.P.M., De Jong Gierveld, J., Van Tilburg, T.G. and Dykstra, P.A. (eds) (1995) *Living Arrangements and Social Networks of Older Adults*. Amsterdam: VU University Press.

Kohli, M., Freter, H.-J., Langehennig, M. *et al.* (1993) *Engagement im Ruhestand. Rentner zwischen Erwerb, Ehrenamt und Hobby*. Opladen.

Kohli, M. and Künemund, H. (1997) *Nachberufliche Tätigkeitsfelder. Konzepte, Forschungslage, Empirie*. Stuttgart: Kohlhammer.

Kohli, M. and Künemund, H. (2000) (eds) *Die zweite Lebenshälfte*. Opladen: Leske & Budrich.

Kohli, M. and Künemund, H. (2001) Partizipation und Engagement älterer Menschen in Deutsches Zentrum für Altersfragen (DZA) (ed.) *Lebenslagen, soziale Ressourcen und gesellschaftliche Integration im Alter*. Opladen: Leske & Budrich.

Kohli, M., Rein, M., Guillemard, A.-M. and Gunsteren, H. (eds) (1991) *Time for Retirement*. Cambridge: Cambridge University Press.

Kohli, M. and Szydlik, M. (ed.) (2000) *Generationen in Familie und Gesellschaft*. Opladen: Leske & Budrich.

Kolland, F. (1996) Kulturwelten der Generationen, in L. Rosenmayr, G. Majce and F. Kolland (eds), *Jahresringe – Altern gestalten*. Wien: Verlag Holzhausen.

Krohne, H.W., Egloff, B., Kohlmann, C.-W. and Tausch, A. (1996) Untersuchungen mit einer deutschen Form der Positive and Negative Affect Schedule (PANAS), *Diagnostica*, 42(2): 139–56.

Kruse, A. (1992) Altersfreundliche Umwelten: Der Beitrag der Technik in P.B. Baltes and J. Mittelstrass (eds) *Altern und gesellschaftliche Entwicklung*. Berlin: deGruyter.

Kruse, A. and Schmitt, E. (1995) Formen der Selbständigkeit in verschiedenen Altersgruppen, *Zeitschrift für Gerontopsychologie und -psychiatrie*, 8: 227–36.

Kruse, A. and Schmitt, E. (1998) Entwicklung von kommunalen Angeboten als Antwort auf die Verschiedenartigkeit von Alternsformen – ein Überblick über die 'Initiative Zweite Lebenshälfte für mehr Lebensqualität', in A. Kruse (ed.) *Psychosoziale Gerontologie. Band 2: Intervention*. Göttingen: Hogrefe.

Kubitschke, L., Hüsing, T., Stähler, B. and Stroetmann, V.N. (2002) *Older Europeans (50+) and Information and Communications Technologies*. Bonn: Empirica.

Kuin, Y., Westerhof, G.J., Dittmann-Kohli, F. and Gerritsen, D. (2001) Psychophysische Integrität und Gesundheitserleben, in F. Dittmann-Kohli, Ch. Bode and G.J. Westerhof (eds) *Die zweite Lebenshälfte – Psychologische Perspektiven*. Stuttgart: Kohlhammer: 343–99.

Künemund, H. (1997) 'Produktive' Tätigkeiten im Alter, in D. Grunow, S. Herkel and H.J. Hummel (eds) *Leistungen und Leistungspotentiale älterer Menschen*, Duisburg: Gerhard-Mercator-Universität und Gesamthochschule Duisburg.

Künemund, H. (2000a) Gesundheit, in M. Kohli and H. Künemund (eds) *Die zweite Lebenshälfte. Gesellschaftliche Lage und Partizipation im Spiegel des Alters-Survey*. Opladen: Leske & Budrich.

Künemund, H. (2000b) Produktive Tätigkeiten, in M. Kohli and H. Künemund (eds) *Die zweite Lebenshälfte*. Opladen: Leske & Budrich.

Küster, C. (1998) Zeitverwendung und Wohnen im Alter in Deutsches Zentrum für Altersfragen (DZA) (ed.) *Wohnbedürfnisse, Zeitverwendung und soziale Netzwerke älterer Menschen*. Frankfurt am Main: Campus: 151–75.

Laczko, F. (1987a) Discouragement, *Unemployment Bulletin*, Issue 24, Summer.

Laczko, F. (1987b) Older workers, unemployment, and the discouraged worker effect, in S. di Gregoria (ed.) *Social Gerontology: New Directions*. London: Croom Helm.

Lago, D. (2000) *Older Women: Key Intergenerational Figures*. http://agexted. cas.psu.edu/docs/21600477.html.

Laicardi, C. and Pezzuti, L. (2000) *Psicologia dell'invecchiamento e della longevità*.

Laicardi, C. and Piperno, A. (1987) *Qualità della vita nella terza età*. Rome: Borla.

Laing & Buisson, (1999) *Care of Elderly People*, Market Survey. London: Laing and Buisson.

Lamura, G., Balducci, C., Melchiorre, M.G. *et al.* (2003) *Comparative Report on Ageing Well and Material Security in Europe*. Report to the European Commission, Centre for Social Policy Research and Development, University of Wales, Bangor.

Lamura, G., Melchiorre, M.G. and Mengani, M. (1999a) Caring for the Caregivers: Challenges for the Italian Social Policy, in *Ageing in a Gendered World*. Santo Domingo: United Nations – INSTRAW.

Lamura, G., Melchiorre, M.G., Quattrini, S. *et al.* (1999b) Reconciliation of work and caring responsibilities. Paper presented at the International Conference 'Active Strategies for an Ageing Workforce', Turku, 12–13 August.

Lamura, G., Melchiorre, M.G., Quattrini, S., Mengani, M. and Albertini, A. (2001) Background report on Italy, in I. Philp (ed.) *Family Care of Older People in Europe*. Amsterdam: IOS Press.

Lang, F.R. and Baltes, M.M. (1997) Brauchen alte Menschen junge Menschen? in L. Krappmann and A. Lepenies (eds) *Alt und Jung: Spannung und Solidarität zwischen den Generationen*. Frankfurt am Main: Campus.

Lang, F.R., Rieckmann, N. and Schwarzer, R. (2000) Lebensqualität über die Lebensspanne, in M. Bullinger, J. Siegrist and U. Ravens-Sieberer (eds) *Lebensqualitätsforschung aus medizinpsychologischer und -soziologischer Perspektive*. Göttingen, Bern: Hogrefe.

Larsen, R. (1978) Thirty years of research on the subjective wellbeing of older Americans, *Journal of Gerontology*, 33: 109–25.

Law n. 448 (2001) Disposizioni per la formazione del bilancio annuale e pluri-ennale dello Stato (law finanziaria 2002), *Gazzetta Ufficiale*, 301, of 29 December (supplemento ordinario).

Law n. 537 (1993) Interventi correttivi di finanza pubblica, *Gazzetta Ufficiale*, 303, of 12 December.

Lazzarini, G. (1994) *Anziani e generazioni*. Milano: Franco Angeli.

Lehr, U. (1994) Die Bedeutung von Aktivität für die Lebensqualität im Alter, in J. Braun, B. Meisheit and S. Trösch (eds) *Aktives Leben im Alter*. Köln: ISAB: 75–83.

Lehr, U. (1997) Gesundheit und Lebensqualität im Alter, *Zeitschrift für Gerontopsychologie und -psychiatrie*, 10(4): 277–87.

Lehr, U. (2000) *Psychologie des Alterns*. Wiebelsheim: Quelle & Meyer.

Lehr, U. and Minnemann, E. (1987) Veränderung von Quantität und Qualität sozialer Kontakte vom 7. bis 9. Lebensjahrzehnt, in U. Lehr and H. Thomae (eds) *Formen seelischen Alterns*. Stuttgart: Enke.

Lehr, U. and Niederfranke, A. (1991) Pensionierung, in W.D. Oswald, W.M. Herrmann, S. Kanowski, U.M. Lehr and H. Thomae (eds) *Gerontologie*. Stuttgart: Kohlhammer.

Lehr, U. and Thomae, H. (eds) (1987) *Formen seelsichen Alterns*. Stuttgart: Enke.

Lewis, J. and McLaverty, C. (1991) Facing up to the needs of the older man-ager, *Personnel Management*, January: 32–5.

Liefboet, K.C. and De Jong Gierveld, J. (1995) Living Arrangements, Socio-economic Resources and Health, in C.P.M. Knipscheer, J. de Jong Gierveld, T.G. van Tilburg and P.A. Dykstra (eds) *Living Arrangements and Social Networks of Older Adults*. Amsterdam: VU University Press.

Linnemann, M. (1996) *Een eenzaam (s)lot?* Amsterdam: Vrije Universiteit (proefschrift).

Linneman, M. (1999) Eenzaamheid, in H. Buijssen (ed.) *Psychologische hulpverlenening aan ouderen*. Baarn: Intro.

Linnemann, M., van Linschoten, P., Royers, T., Nelissen, H. and Nitsche, B. (2001) *Eenzaam op leeftijd; interventies bij eenzame ouderen*. Utrecht: NIZW.

Livraghi, R. (1996) Le donne anziane in Italia, *OggiDomaniAnziani*, 1: 81–98.

Livraghi, R. (1997) Il concetto di ben-essere e gli anziani in Federazione Nazionale Pensionati CISL (ed.) *Anziani '97 – Tra emarginazio ne e opportunità*. Rome: Edizioni Lavoro.

Love, D. O. and Torrance, W. D. (1989) The impact of worker age on unemployment and earnings after plant closings, *Journal of Gerontology: Social Sciences*, 44(5): 190–5.

Luciani, E. (1999) Associazionismo virtuale nella terza età, in *Federazione Nazionale Pensionati CISL (a cura di) Anziani '98 – Tra uguaglianza e diversità. Secondo rapporto sulla condizione della persona anziana*. Rome: Edizioni Lavoro.

Luciani, E. (2000) Opportunità in rete in Federazione Nazionale Pensionati CISL (ed.) *Anziani '99–2000 – L'integrazione possibile*. Rome: Edizioni Lavoro.

Maas, I.A.M., Gijsen, R., Lobbezoo, I.E. and Poos, M.J.J.C. (eds) (1997) Volksgezondheid toekomst verkenning 1997, I. De gezondheidstoestand: een actualisering, Maarssen/Bilthoven: Elsevier/De Tijdstroom/RIVM.

Maes, B. and Petry, K. (2000) Naar een groeiende concensus over de betekenis van het concept kwaliteit van leven, *Tijdschr voor Orthopedagogiek*, 39(12): 27–40.

Magnusson, L., Hanson, E., Berthold, H., Andersson, B. and Johansson, C. (2001) *Stöd till äldre och*. Uppsala: Uppsala universitet, Sociologiska institutionen.

Mahoney, F.I. and Barthel, D.W. (1965) Functional evaluation: the Barthel Index, *Maryland State Medical Journal*, 14: 61–5.

Maier, G. (2000) Zwischen Arbeit und Ruhestand, in H.-W. Wahl and C. Tesch-Römer (eds) *Angewandte Gerontologie in Schlüsselbegriffen*, Stuttgart: Kohlhammer.

Marbach, J.H. (2001) Aktionsraum und soziales Netzwerk: Reichweite und Ressourcen der Lebensführung im Alter, *Zeitschrift für Gerontologie und Geriatrie*, 34(4): 319–26.

Marcellini, F., Gaglirdi, C., Leonardi, F. and Spazzafumo, L. (1999) *Mobilità e qualità della vita degli anziani*. Milano: Franco Angeli.

Marmot, M., Banks, J., Blundell, R., Lessof, C. and Nazroo, J. (2003) *Health, Wealth and Lifestyles of the Older Population in England: The 2002 English Longitudinal Study of Ageing*. London: Institute for Fiscal Studies,

Martin, M. (2001) *Verfügbarkeit und Nutzung menschlicher Ressourcen im Alter*. Idstein: Schulz-Kirchner Verlag.

Martin, P. (2000) Ergebnisse zur Bedeutung 'aktiven' Alterns in H.-W. Wahl and C. Tesch-Römer (eds) *Angewandte Gerontologie in Schlüsselbegriffen*. Stuttgart: Kohlhammer.

Martin, P., Ettrich, K.U., Lehr, U. et al. (eds) (2000) *Aspekte der Entwicklung im mittleren und höheren Lebensalter*. Darmstadt: Steinkopff.

Mathwig, G. and Mollenkopf, H. (1996) Ältere Menschen: Problem- und Wohlfahrtslagen, in W. Zapf and R. Habich (eds) *Wohlfahrtsentwicklung im vereinten Deutschland*. Berlin: Edition Sigma.

Maule, A.J., Cliff, D.R. and Taylor, R. (1996) Early retirement decisions and how they affect later quality of life, *Ageing and Society*, 16: 177–204.

Mayer, K.U. and Baltes, P.B. (eds) (1996) *Die Berliner Altersstudie*. Berlin: Akademie-Verlag.

Mayer, K.U. and Wagner, M. (1996) Lebenslagen und soziale Ungleichheit im hohen Alter, in K.U. Mayer and P.B. Baltes (eds) *Die Berliner Altersstudie*. Berlin: Akademie-Verlag.

Mayring, P. (1987) Subjektives Wohlbefinden im Alter, *Zeitschrift für Gerontologie*, 20: 367–76.

Mayring, P. (1991) Die Erfassung subjektiven Wohlbefindens, in A. Abele and P. Becker (eds) *Wohlbefinden: Theorie, Empirie, Diagnostik*. Munich: Juventa.

Mayring, P. (2000) Pensionierung als Krise oder Glücksgewinn? Ergebnisse aus einer quantitativ-qualitativen Längsschnittuntersuchung, *Zeitschrift für Gerontologie und Geriatrie*, 33(2): 124–33.

McGoldrick, A. and Cooper, C. (1998) *Early Retirement*. Aldershot: Gower.

McKay, S. and Middleton, S. (1998) *Characteristics of Older Workers*. London: HMSO.

Meier, D. (1995) Lebensqualität im Alter. Eine Studie zur Erfassung der individuellen Lebensqualität von gesunden Älteren, von Patienten im Anfangsstadium einer Demenz und ihren Angehörigen. Bern, Berlin, Frankfurt am Main: Lang.

Melchiorre M.G., Sirolla C., Quattrini S., Lamura G. (2001) Elderly care and respite services, *Gerontology, International Journal of Experimental, Clinical and Behavioural Gerontology*, 47 (suppl 1): 159.

Mengani, M., Lamura, G., and Melchiorre, M.G. (1999) *L'assistenza famigliare agli anziani*. Ancona: Il Lavoro Editoriale.

Meyer, S. and Schulze, E. (1996) Ein neuer Sprung der technischen Entwicklung, in S. Gräbe (ed.) *Vernetzte Technik für private Haushalte*. Frankfurt am Main: Campus.

Meyer, S., Schulze, E. and Müller, P. (1997) *Das intelligente Haus*. Frankfurt am Main: Campus.

Midwinter, E. (1991) *The British Gas Report on Attitudes to Ageing*. London: British Gas.

Miniati, S. (2000) Lavoro e pensione: un rapporto da disegnare, in G. Geroldi (ed.) *Lavorare da anziani e da pensionati*. Milano: Franco Angeli.

Ministerie van Volkshuisvesting en Ruimtelijke ordening (2000) *Volkshuisvesting in cijfers*. Den Haag: Ministerie VROM.

Ministerie van Volksgezondheid, Welzijn en sport (1999) *Welzijnsnota 1999–2002*. Den Haag: Ministerie VWS.

Ministero dell'Interno – Direzione Generale dei Servizi Civili (1994) *La famiglia anziana*. Rome: Indagine Istiss.

Minkler, M. and Estes, C. (1999) (eds) *Critical Gerontology: Perspectives from Political and Moral Economy*. Amityville, NY: Baywood.

Minnemann, E. (1992) Soziale Beziehungen älterer Menschen, in A. Niederfranke, U.M. Lehr, F. Oswald and G. Maier (eds) *Altern in unserer Zeit*. Wiesbaden: Quelle & Meyer.

Minnemann, E. (1994a) *Die Bedeutung sozialer Beziehungen für Lebenszufriedenheit im Alter*. Regensburg: Roderer.

Minnemann, E. (1994b) Geschlechtsspezifische Unterschiede der Gestaltung sozialer Beziehungen im Alter, *Zeitschrift für Gerontologie*, 27(1): 33–41.

Mirabile, M.L. and Carrera, F. (1999) La Seconda Carriera, *Rassegna Sindacale*, supplement to no. 5.

Mirabile, M.L., Carrera, F. and Tomassini, C. (1998) *Oltre i 45 anni. Programma Leonardo Da Vinci*. Rome: IESS-AE.

Mollenkopf, H. (1998) Technik im Dienste der Lebensqualität im Alter in P. Borscheid, H. Bausinger and L. Rosenmayr (eds) *Die Gesellschaft braucht die Alten*. Opladen: Leske & Budrich.

Mollenkopf, H. and Flaschenträger, P. (1996) *Mobilität zur sozialen Teilhabe im Alter*. Berlin: WZB.

Mollenkopf, H. and Hampel, J. (1994) *Technik, Alter, Lebensqualität*. Schriftenreihe des Bundesministeriums für Familie und Senioren, Band 23. Stuttgart: Kohlhammer.

Mollenkopf, H., Mix, S., Gäng, K. and Kwon, S. (2001) Alter und Technik, in Deutsches Zentrum für Altersfragen (DZA) (ed.) *Personale, gesundheitliche und Umweltressourcen im Alter*, Band 1. Opladen: Leske & Budrich.

Monzeglio, E. (1996) Tecnologie costruttive, accessibilità e sicurezza nella organizzazione spaziale delle Residenze Sanitarie Assistenziali, *Gerontechnology*, 3–4: 69–79.

Motel, A. (2000) Einkommen und Vermögen in M. Kohli and H. Künemund (eds) *Die zweite Lebenshälfte*. Opladen: Leske & Budrich.

Motel, A., Künemund, H. and Bode, Ch. (2000) Wohnen und Wohnumfeld, in M. Kohli and H. Künemund (eds) *Die zweite Lebenshälfte*. Opladen: Leske & Budrich.

Moyer, M.S. (1992) Sibling relationships among older adults, *Generations*, 16(3): 55–8.

Mulder, A. (2001) Verhuizen is geen pretje, in Nirov *Discussiedagen Bouwen en Wonen* 2001 (Volume Nirov Conference Papers). Den Haag: Nirov: 23–30.

Münnich, M. and Illgen, M. (1999) Ausstattung privater Haushalte mit langlebigen Gebraushsgütern, *Wirtschaft und Statistik* 1: 46–54.

Myers, R. (1983) More about the controversy on early retirement, *Ageing and Work*, 5: 83–91.

Naegele, G. (1992) *Zwischen Arbeit und Rente*. Augsburg: Maro.

Naegele, G. (1998) Lebenslagen älterer Menschen, in A. Kruse (ed.) *Psychosoziale Gerontologie. Band 1: Grundlagen*. Göttingen: Hogrefe.

Naegele, G. (2000) Finanzielle Absicherung und Armut im Alter, in H.-W. Wahl and C. Tesch-Römer (eds) *Angewandte Gerontologie in Schlüsselbegriffen*. Stuttgart: Kohlhammer.

Naegele, G. and Frerichs, F. (1996) Situation und Perspektiven der Alterserwerbsarbeit in der Bundesrepublik Deutschland, *Aus Politik und Zeitgeschichte*, 35: 33–45.

Nazroo, J., Bajekal, M., Blane, D., Grewal, I. and Lewis, J. (2003) *Ethnic Inequalities in Quality of Life at Older Ages: Subjective and Objective Components*. Sheffield: Growing Older Programme, University of Sheffield.

Niederfranke, A. (1991) *Neue Chancen nach der Lebensmitte – Spurwechsel?* Stuttgart: Ministerium für Arbeit, Gesundheit, Familie und Frauen Baden-Württemberg.

Niederfranke, A. (1992) *Ältere Frauen in der Auseinandersetzung mit Berufsaufgabe und Partnerverlust*. Stuttgart: Kohlhammer.

Niederfranke, A. (1996) Nachberufliche Tätigkeiten – Wunsch oder Wirklichkeit? *Zeitschrift für Gerontologie und Geriatrie*, 29(5): 362–6.

Niehörster, G., Garms-Homolova, V. and Varenhorst, V. (1998) *Identifizierung von Potentialen für eine selbständigere Lebensführung*. Schriftenreihe des BFSFJ, Band 147, 4. Stuttgart: Kohlhammer.

Niepel, T. (1995) *Effektivität und Effizienz von Beratung zur Wohnungsanpassung. Bericht im Auftrag des Ministeriums für Arbeit, Gesundheit und Soziales des Landes Nordrhein-Westfalen*. Bielefeld: Eigenverlag.

Nimwegen, N. and Moors, H. (1997) *Population Ageing and Policy Options*. Working paper. The Hague: NIDI.

Nisenson, L.G., Pepper, C.M., Schwenk, T.L. and Coyne, J.C. (1988) The nature and prevalence of anxiety disorders in primary care, *General Hospital Psychiatrics*, 20: 21–8.

Nocon, A. and Peace, N. (1999) Sheltered Housing and Community Care, *Social Policy and Administration*, 33(2): 164–80.

Noll, H. (1997) Wohlstand, Lebensqualität und Wohlbefinden in den Ländern der Europäischen Union, in S. Hradil and S. Immerfall (eds) *Die Westeuropäischen Gesellschaften im Vergleich*. Opladen: Leske & Budrich.

Noll, H. (2000) *The European System of Social Indicators*. Mannheim: ZUMA.

Noll, H. and Schöb, A. (2002) Lebensqualität im Alter in Deutsches Zentrum für Altersfragen (DZA) (ed.) *Expertisen zum 4, Band 1: Konzepte, Forschungsfelder, Lebensqualität*. Hannover: Vincentz.

O'Boyle, C., McGee, H., Hickey, A., Joyce, C. and O'Malley, K. (1993) *The Schedule for the Evaluation of Individual Quality of Life*. Dublin: Department of Psychology, Royal College of Surgeons in Ireland.

OECD (1996) *Caring for Frail Elderly People: Policies in Evolution*. Paris: OECD.

OECD (2000) *Health Data 2000*. Paris: OECD.

OECD (2001a) *Ageing and Income*. Paris: OECD.

OECD (2001b) *Understanding the Digital Divide*. Paris: OECD.

Oeuppen, J. and Vaupel, J. (2002) Broken limits to life expectancy, *Science*, 296: 1–2.

Olbrich, E. (1995) Möglichkeiten und Grenzen selbständiger Lebensführung im Alter – Einführung und Überblick, *Zeitschrift für Gerontopsychologie und -psychiatrie*, 8(4): 183–98.

Olbrich, E. (1996) Menschengerechte Umweltgestaltung, *Zeitschrift für Gerontologie und Geriatrie*, 29(4): 257–66.

Oldman, C. (2000) *Blurring the Boundaries: A Fresh Look at Housing and Care Provision for Older People*. York: Joseph Rowntree Foundation.

Olini, G. (1999) Anziani, tempo di vita, tempo di lavoro in Federazione Nazionale Pensionati CISL (ed.) *Anziani '98 – Tra uguaglianza e diversità*. Rome: Edizioni Lavoro.

Oppikofer, S., Albrecht, K., Schelling, H.R. and Wettstein, A. (2002) Die Auswirkungen sozialer Unterstützung auf das Wohlbefinden dementer Heimbewohnerinnen und Heimbewohner, *Zeitschrift für Gerontologie und Geriatrie*, 35(1): 39–48.

Oswald, F., Schmitt, M., Gansera-Baumann, B., Martin, M. and Sperling, U. (2000) *Subjektive Wohnbedeutungen und Veränderungen im Wohnbereich*. Heidelberg: DZFA.

Oswald, W.D., Hagen, B. and Rupprecht, R. (1998) Bedingungen der Erhaltung und Förderung von Selbständigkeit im höheren Lebensalter (SIMA) – Teil X: Verlaufsanalyse des kognitiven Status, *Zeitschrift für Gerontopsychologie und -psychiatrie*, 11(4): 202–21.

Pace, R. (1996) Reti formali ed informali di assistenza agli anziani: risultati di un'indagine pilota in Puglia, in *Politiche familiari, welfare e sviluppo sostenibile*. Rome: IRP-CNR.

Paciaroni, E. (2000) *Telemedicina*. Ancona: INRCA – Il Lavoro Editoriale.

Pacolet, J. and Bouten, R. (2000) *Social Protection for Dependency in Old Age*. Leuten: HIVA.

Palomba, R., Misiti, M. and Sabatino, D. (eds) (2001) La vecchiaia può attendere. IRP- CNR, *Collana Quaderni Demotrends*, 1 March.

Peace, S. and Holland, C. (2001a) *Inclusive Housing in an Ageing Society*. Southampton: Policy Press.

Peace, S. and Holland, C. (2001b) Homely residential care: a contradiction in terms? *Journal of Social Policy*, 30(3): 393–410.

Peace, S., Holland, C. and Kellaher, L. (2003) *Environment and Identity in Later Life: a Cross-setting Study*. Sheffield: Growing Older Programme, University of Sheffield.

Peace, S., Kellaher, L. and Willcocks, D. (1997) *Re-evaluating Residential Care*. Buckingham: Open University Press.

Pellegrino, M. (2000) *Aiutare chi aiuta*. Rome: Edizioni Lavoro.

Penninx, B.W.J.H. (1994) Social Support and Social Network among Elderly with Joint Disorders in D.J.H. Deeg and M. Westendorp-de Serriere (eds), *Autonomy and Wellbeing in the Aging Population I*. Amsterdam: Thela-Thesis.

Penninx, K. (1999) *De buurt voor alle leeftijden*. Utrecht: NIZW Uitgeverij.

Penninx, B.W.J.H., Leveille, S., Ferruci, L. *et al.* (1999) Exploring the effect of depression on physical disability: longitudinal evidence from the established population for epidemiological studies for the elderly, *American Journal of Public Health* 89(9): 1346–52.

Percival, J. (2001) Self-esteem and social motivation in age-segregated settings, *Housing Studies*, 16(6): 827–40.

Persson, G., Boström, G. Allebäck, P. *et al.* (2001) Elderly people's health – 65 and after. *Scandinavian Journal of Public Health*, (Suppl 58), 29: 117–31.

275

Phillipson, C. and Walker, A. (1986) (eds) *Ageing and Social Policy*, London: Gower.

Phillipson, C. and Walker, A. (1987) The Case for a Critical Gerontology, in S. de Gregario (ed.) *Social Gerontology: New Directions*, London: Gower.

Philp, I. (ed) (2001) *Family Care of Older People in Europe*. Amsterdam: IOS Press.

Piachaud, D. (1986) Disability, retirement and unemployment of older men, *Journal of Social Policy*, 15(2): 145–62.

Pierpaoli, P. (2002) La minima dell'Inps, *Corriere Adriatico*, 3 February: 11.

Platman, K. and Tinker, A. (1998) Getting on in the BBC: a case study of older workers, *Ageing and Society*, 18: 513–35.

Pohlmann, S. (2001) *Das Altern der Gesellschaft als globale Herausforderung – Deutsche Impulse*. Schriftenreihe des BFSFJ, Band 201. Stuttgart: Kohlhammer.

Pot, A.M., and Deeg, D.J.H. (1997) De gezondheidstoestand van ouderen, in J.P. Mackenbach and H. Verkleij (eds) *Volksgezondheid toekomst verkenning 1997; II Gezondheidsverschillen*. Bilthoven/Maarssen: Rijksinstituut voor volksgezondheid en milieu/Elsevier/De Tijdstroom.

Presidenza del Consiglio dei Ministri (2000) *Relazione biennale al Parlamento sulla condizione dell'anziano 1998–1999*. Rome: Dipartimento per gli Affari Social.

Qureshi, H. and Henwood, M. (2000) *Older People's Definitions of Quality Services*. York: Joseph Rowntree Foundation.

Ramakers, C. and Miltenburg, T. van (1998) *Persoonsgebonden budge*. Nijmegen: ITS.

Ranieri, P., Di Niro, M.G., Manes Gravina, E. et al. (2000) Benessere psico-sociale in anziani ospiti di RSA, *Giornale di Gerontologia*, 11: 807.

Ravens-Sieberer, U. and Cieza, A. (eds) (2000) *Lebensqualität und Gesundheitsökonomie in der Medizin: Konzepte, Methoden, Anwendung*. Landsberg: Ecomed.

Raynes, N., Temple, B. Clenister, C. and Coulthard, L. (2001) *Getting Older People's Views on Quality Home Care Services*. York: Joseph Rowntree Foundation.

Regione Veneto (2002) *Il Progetto Regionale*. www.osservareperconoscere.it.

Renzi, C., Pavan, R., Ulisse, M. and Marcellini F. (1995) *Rilevazione della popolazione anziana e dei servizi socio-assistenziali dedicati.* Ancona: INRCA – Regione Marche.

Rietz, C. and Rudinger, G. (2000) Aspekte der subjektiven und objektiven Lebensqualität, in P. Martin, K.U. Ettrich, U. Lehr et al. (eds) *Aspekte der Entwicklung im mittleren und höheren Lebensalter.* Darmstadt: Steinkopff.

RMO-advies (1997) *Vereenzaming in de samenleving.* Rijswijk: RMO.

Robertson, I., Warr, P., Butcher, V., Callinan, M. and Bardzil, P. (2003) *Older People's Experience of Paid Employment: Participation and Quality of Life.* Sheffield: Growing Older Programme, University of Sheffield.

Rogerson, R.J., Findlay, A.M., Coombes, M.G. and Morris, A. (1989) Indicators of quality of life, *Environment and Planning,* 21: 1655–66.

Romano, M.C. and Sgritta, G.B. (2000) La sfida della terza età nella società post-tradizionale, in Federazione Nazionale Pensionati CISL (ed.) *Anziani '99–2000 – L'integrazione possibile.* Rome: Edizioni Lavoro.

Ronström, O. (2002) The making of older immigrants in Sweden, in L. Andersson (ed.) *Cultural Gerontology.* Westport, CT: Auburn House/ Greenwood Publishing Group.

Rosenbladt, B. von (ed.) (2000) *Freiwilliges Engagement in Deutschland.* Band 1: Gesamtbericht. Schriftenerihe des BFSFJ, Band 194.1. Stuttgart: Kohlhammer.

Rosenblum, M. (1975) The last push: from discouraged worker to involuntary retirement, *Industrial Gerontology,* 2: 14–22.

Rosenmayer, L. and Kockeis, E. (1963) Propositions for a sociological theory of ageing and the family, *International Social Service Journal,* 15(3): 410–26.

Rothermund, K. and Brandstädter, J. (1998) Auswirkungen von Belastungen und Verlusten auf die Lebensqualität: alters- und lebenszeitgebundene Moderationseffekte, *Zeitschrift für Klinische Psychologie,* 27(2): 86–92.

Rothermund, K., Dillmann, U. and Brandtstädter, J. (1994) Belastende Lebenssituationen im mittleren und höheren Erwachsenenalter: Zur differen- tiellen Wirksamkeit assimilativer und akkomodativer Bewältigung, *Zeitschrift für Gesundheitspsychologie,* 2(4): 245–68.

Rowe, J. and Kahn, R. (1997) The forum – successful ageing, *The Gerontologist,* 37(4): 433–40.

Rudinger, G. (1996) Alter und Technik, *Zeitschrift für Gerontologie und Geriatrie*, 29(4): 243–56.

Rudinger, G., Espey, J., Neur, H. and Simon, U. (1991) *Abschlussbericht zum Projekt 'Alter und Technik' (ALTEC)*. Bonn: Psychologisches Institut, Universität Bonn.

Rudinger, G., Rietz, Ch. and Schiffhorst, G. (1997) Aspekte der subjektiven und objektiven Lebensqualität, *Zeitschrift für Gerontopsychologie und -psychiatrie*, 10(4): 259–75.

Santanera, F., Breda, M.G. and Dalmazio, F. (1994) *Anziani malati cronici*. Torino: UTET Libreria.

Saup, W. (1991) *Konstruktives Altern: Ein Beitrag zum Altern von Frauen aus entwicklungspsychologischer Sicht*. Göttingen: Hogrefe.

Saup, W. and Mayring, P. (1995) Pensionierung, in R. Oerter and L. Montada (eds) *Entwicklungspsychologie: Ein Lehrbuch, 3*. Auflage. Weinheim: Beltz, PVU.

Saup, W. and Schröppel, H. (1993) *Wenn Altenheimbewohner selbst bestimmen*. Augsburg: Verlag für Psychologie.

Schaeffer, D. (1999) Care Management. *Zeitschrift für Gesundheitswissenschaften*, 7(3): 233–51.

Scharf, T., Phillipson, C., Smith, A. and Kingston, P. (2003) *Older People in Deprived Neighbourhoods: Social Exclusion and Quality of Life in Old Age*. Sheffield: Growing Older Programme, University of Sheffield.

Scharf, T., Van der Meer, M., Thissen, F. and Melchiorre, M.G. (2003) *Contextualising Adult Wellbeing in Europe*. Report to European Commission, Centre for Social Policy Research and Development, University of Wales, Bangor.

Scheewe, P. (1996) Wohnverhältnisse älterer Menschen, *Wirtschaft und Statistik*, 4: 228–38.

Schena, F., Martinelli, C. and Noro, G. (2000) Il significato dell'attività fisica nell'anziano istituzionalizzato, *Giornale di Gerontologia*, 9: 597–607.

Schmitt, E. (2001) Zur Bedeutung von Erwerbstätigkeit und Arbeitslosigkeit im mittleren und höheren Erwachsenenalter für das subjektive Alterserleben und die Wahrnehmung von Potentialen und Barrieren eines mitverantwortlichen Lebens, *Zeitschrift für Gerontologie und Geriatrie*, 34(3): 218–31.

Schmitt, E., Kruse, A. and Olbrich, E. (1994) Wohnen im Alter – Zusammenhänge zwischen Selbständigkeit und Qualität des Wohnumfeldes, *Zeitschrift für Gerontologie*, 27: 390–8.

Schneekloth, U. and Müller, U. (1997) *Hilfe- und Pflegebedürftige in Heimen. Endbericht zur Repräsentativerhebung im Forschungsprojekt 'Möglichkeiten und Grenzen selbständiger Lebensführung in Einrichtungen'*. Stuttgart: Kohlhammer.

Schneekloth, U. and Müller, U. (2000) *Wirkungen der Pflegeversicherung. Schriftenreihe des Bundesministeriums für Gesundheit*. Band 127, Baden-Baden: Nomos Verlag.

Schneider, H.D. (1995) Die soziale Umwelt im Alter als Ressource oder als Belastung? in A. Kruse and R. Schmitz-Scherzer (eds) *Psychologie der Lebensalter*. Darmstadt: Steinkopff.

Schölzel-Dorenbos, C.J.M. (2000) Meting van kwaliteit van leven van patiënten met dementie van het Alzheimertype en hun verzorgers, *Tijdschrift voor Gerontologie en Geriatrie*, 31(1): 23–7.

Schröder, H. (1995) Materiell gesichert, aber häufig isoliert. Zur Lebenssituation älterer Menschen im vereinten Deutschland, *Informationsdienst Soziale Indikatoren*, 13: 11–15.

Schulze, G. (1994) Das Projekt des schönen Lebens, in A. Bellebaum and K. Barheier (eds) *Lebensqualität*. Opladen: Westdeutscher Verlag.

Schumacher, J., Klaiberg, A. and Brähler, E. (eds) (2003) *Diagnostische Verfahren zu Lebensqualität und Wohlbefinden*. Göttingen: Hogrefe.

Schumacher, J., Wilz, G. and Brähler, E. (1997) Zum Einfluss dispositioneller Bewältigungsstrategien auf Körperbeschwerden und Lebenszufriedenheit im Alter, *Zeitschrift für Gerontologie und Geriatrie*, 30(5): 338–47.

Schwarzer, R. and Koll, N. (2001) Personale Ressourcen im Alter in Deutsches Zentrum für Altersfragen (DZA) (ed.) *Personale, gesundheitliche und Umweltressourcen im Alter*, Band I. Opladen: Leske & Budrich.

Schwitzer, K.-P. (1995) Ungleichheit und Angleichung von Lebensverhältnissen im vereinten Deutschland am Beispiel älterer Menschen, in W. Glatzer and H.-H. Noll (eds) *Getrennt vereint: Lebensverhältnisse in Deutschland seit der Wiedervereinigung*. Frankfurt am Main: Campus.

SCP (2001) *De Sociale staat van Nederland*. Den Haag: Sociaal Cultureel Planbureau.

Seifert, W. (1996) Einwanderungsland Deutschland, in W. Zapf and R. Habich (eds) *Wohlfahrtsentwicklung im vereinten Deutschland*. Berlin: Edition Sigma.

Sen, A. (1993) *Il tenore di vita tra benessere e libertà*. Venice: Marsilio.

Seniorweb (2000) *Annual Report*. Utrecht: Seniorweb.

SER (1999) *Gezondheidszorg in het licht van de toekomstige vergrijzing*. Den Haag: SER.

Sgadari, A., Tarsitani, P., Venturiero, V. *et al.* (2000) Antidepressivi e rischio di cadute e frattura di femore negli anziani istituzionalizzati, *Giornale di Gerontologia*, 6: 366–7.

Sgritta, G.B. and Saporiti, A. (1997) *La staffetta anziani e giovan*. Rome: Edizioni Lavoro.

Sgritta, G.B. and Saporiti, A. (1998) Gli anziani e il volontariato, *OggiDomaniAnziani*, 1: 11–75.

Sheldon, J.H. (1948) *The Social Medicine of Old Age*. Oxford: Oxford University Press.

Silveira, E. and Allebeck, P. (2001) Migration, ageing and mental health: an ethnographic study on perceptions of life satisfaction, anxiety and depression in older Somali men in east London, *International Journal of Social Welfare*, 10: 309–20.

Sixsmith, A, (1994) New technology and community care, *Health and Social Care*, 2: 367–78.

Smith, J. and Baltes, P.B. (1996) Altern aus psychologischer Perspektive: Trends und Profile im hohen Alter, in K.U. Mayer and P.B. Baltes (eds) *Die Berliner Altersstudie*. Berlin: Akademie-Verlag.

Smith, J., Fleeson, W., Geiselmann, B., Settersten, R. and Kunzmann, U. (1996) Wohlbefinden im hohen Alter, in K.U. Mayer and P.B. Baltes (eds) *Die Berliner Altersstudie*. Berlin: Akademie-Verlag.

Socci, M., Melchiorre, M.G., Quattrini, S. and Lamura, G. (2003) Elderly care provided by foreign immigrants, *Generations Review (Journal of the British Society of Gerontology)*, 13(4): 9–13.

Socci, M., Melchiorre, M.G., Quattrini, S., Sirolla, C. and Lamura, G. (2001) L'assistenza domiciliare agli anziani fornita da personale immigrato, *Prospettive Sociali e Sanitarie*, 13: 12–16.

Sociaal Cultureel Planbureau (1997) *Rapportage Ouderen 1996*. Den Haag: SCP.

Sociaal Cultureel Planbureau (1999) *Rapportage Ouderen 1998*. Den Haag: SCP.

Sociaal Cultureel Planbureau (2001) *Rapportage Ouderen 2001*. Den Haag: SCP.

Social Statutes XI – SGB XI. *Soziale Pflegeversicherung*, 5th edn. Munich: C.H. Beck.

SOU 2001: 48 (2001) Att vara med på riktigt. Betänkande av Kommundemokratikommittén, Stockholm: Fritzes.

SOU 2002: 15 (2002) IT och äldre. IT-kommissionens rapport 2/2002, Stockholm: Fritzes.

SOU 2002: 29 (2002) Riv ålderstrappan! Livslopp i förändring. Diskussionsbetänkande av den parlamentariska äldreberedningen Senior 2005, Stockholm: Fritzes.

Sowarka, D. (2000) Merkmale der Lebensqualität in Pflegeeinrichtungen, in H. Entzian, K.I. Giercke, Th. Kie and R. Schmidt (eds) *Soziale Gerontologie*. Frankfurt am Main: Mabuse-Verlag.

SPI-CGIL (1990) *Dall'assistenzialismo ai nuovi diritti*. Rome: EdiSpi.

SPI-CGIL/CER (1997) *Gli anziani in Italia. VI° Rapporto*. Rome: Ediesse.

Spruytte, N., Verschueren, K. and Marcoen, A. (1999) Grootouders : hun beleving van de relatie met het oudste kleinkind en hun welbevinden, *Tijdschrift voor Gerontologie en Geriatrie*, 30(1): 21–30.

Statistics Sweden (2000) *Living conditions of the elderly 1980–1998*, Statistics Sweden, Örebro: Socialdepartementet, Socialstyrelsen.

Staudinger, U.M. (2000) Viele Gründe sprechen dagegen, und trotzdem geht es vielen Menschen gut: Das Paradox des subjektiven Wohlbefindens, *Psychologische Rundschau*, 51(4): 185–97.

Staudinger, U.M. and Freund, A. (1998) Krank und 'arm' im hohen Alter und trotzdem guten Mutes? *Zeitschrift für Klinische Psychologie*, 27(2): 78–85.

Staudinger, U.M. and Greve, W. (2001) Resilienz im Alter, in Deutsches Zentrum für Altersfragen (DZA) (ed.) *Personale, gesundheitliche und Umweltressourcen im Alter*, Band 1. Opladen: Leske & Budrich.

Staudinger, U.M., Freund, A., Linden, M. and Maas, I. (1996) Selbst, Persönlichkeit und Lebensgestaltung: Psychologische Widerstandsfähigkeit und Vulnerabilität, in K.U. Mayer and P.B. Baltes (eds) *Die Berliner Altersstudie*. Berlin: Akademie Verlag.

Steinwachs, K.C., Oswald, W.D., Hagen, B. and Rupprecht, R. (1998) Bedingungen der Erhaltung und Förderung von Selbständigkeit im höheren Lebensalter (SIMA), *Zeitschrift für Gerontopsychologie und -psychiatrie*, 11(4): 222–39.

Stevens, N. (1997) Vriendschap als sleutel tot welbevinden: een cursus voor vrowwen boven de 55 jaar. Tijdschrift voor Gerontologie en Geriatrie, 28, 18–26.

Steverink, N. and Timmer, E. (2001) Das subjektive Alterserleben, in F. Dittmann-Kohli, Ch. Bode and G.J. Westerhof (eds) *Die zweite Lebenshälfte*. Schriftenreihe des BFSFJ Band 195. Stuttgart: Kohlhammer.

Sticker, E.J. (1987) Beziehungen zwischen Grosseltern und Enkeln. *Zeitschrift für Gerontologie*, 20(5): 269–74.

Stolarz, H. (1997) *10 Jahre Wohnungsanpassung in Deutschland*. KDA-Schriftenreihe Forum Nr 32. Köln: Kuratorium Deutsche Altershilfe.

Styrborn, K. (1997) Äldres komplexa vårdbehov. Rapport 1997: 11. Stockholms Läns Äldrecentrum 11. Stockholm: Gerontology Research Center.

Szebehely, M. (1999) Concepts and trends in home care for frail elderly people in France and in Sweden, in *Comparing Social Welfare Systems in Nordic Europe and France*. Paris: MIRE.

Szydlik, M. (2000) *Lebenslange Solidarität? Generationenbeziehungen zwischen erwachsenen Kindern und Eltern*. Opladen: Leske & Budrich.

Tanner, D. (2001) Sustaining the self in later life: supporting older people in the community, *Ageing and Society*, 21: 255–78.

Taylor, P. and Walker, A. (1991) *Too Old at 50*. London: Campaign for Work.

Taylor, P. and Walker, A. (1996) Intergenerational relations in employment, in A. Walker (ed.) *The New Generational Contract*. London: UCL Press.

Teipen, Ch. and Zierep, E. (1996) Konsensuelle und konfliktorische Frühverrentung, *Zeitschrift für Gerontologie und Geriatrie*, 29(5): 334–8.

Teng, B. (2001) Relevant en woonzorgzones, in Nirov *Discussiedagen Bouwen en Wonen* 2001. (Volume Nirov Conference Papers) Den Haag: Nirov: 61–6.

Tesch-Römer, C. (1998) Alltagsaktivitäten und Tagesstimmungen im Alter, *Zeitschrift für Gerontologie und Geriatrie*, 31: 257–62.

Tesch-Römer, C. (2000) Einsamkeit, in H.-W. Wahl and C. Tesch-Römer (eds) *Angewandte Gerontologie in Schlüsselbegriffen*. Stuttgart: Kohlhammer.

Tesch-Römer, C., von Kondratowitz, H.J, and Motel-Klingebiel, A. (2001) Quality of life in the context of intergenerational solidarity, in S.O. Daatland and K. Herlofson (eds) *Ageing, Intergenerational Relations, Care Systems and Quality of Life.* Oslo: Nova: 63–73.

Tews, H.P. (1993) Altern Ost – Altern West: Ergebnisse zum deutsch-deutschen Vergleich, in G. Naegele and H.P. Tews (eds) *Lebenslagen im Strukturwandel des Alters.* Opladen: Westdeutscher Verlag.

Thomae, H. (1987) Alternsformen: Wege zu ihrer methodischen und begrif-flichen Erfassung, in U. Lehr and H. Thomae (eds) *Formen seelischen Alterns.* Stuttgart: Enke.

Thomae, H. (1994) Trust, social support, and relying on others, *Zeitschrift für Gerontologie,* 27: 103–9.

Tilburg, T.G. (1995) Delineation of the social network and differences in network size, in C.P.M. Knipscheer, J. de Jong Gierveld, T.G. van Tilburg and P.A. Dykstra (eds) *Living Arrangements and Social Networks of Older Adults.* Amsterdam: VU University Press.

Tillsley, C. (1995) Older workers: findings from the 1994 Labour Force Survey, *Employment Gazette,* April.

Tomassini, C., Glaser, K., Wolf, D.A., Broese van Groenou, M.I. and Grundy, E. (2004) Living arrangements among older people, *Population Trends,* 115, Spring: 24–35.

Töpfer, A.-K., Strosberg, M. and Oswald, W.D. (1998) Bedingungen der Erhaltung und Förderung von Selbständigkeit im höheren Lebensalter (SIMA). Teil VIII: Soziale Integration, Soziale Netzwerke und Soziale Unterstützung, *Zeitschrift für Gerontopsychologie und Psychiatrie,* 11(3): 139–58.

Torgén, M., Stenlund, C., Ahlberg, G. and Marklund, S. (2001) *Ett hållbart arbetsliv för alla åldrar.* Rapport 2001: 01, Stockholm. Arbetslivsinstitutet, (National Institute for Working Life).

Tornstam, L. (1989) Gerotranscendence: a reformulation of the disengage-ment theory, *Aging: Clinical and Experimental Research,* 1(1): 55–63.

Tornstam, L. (1997) Gerotranscendence in a broad cross-sectional perspective, *Journal of Aging and Identity,* 2(1): 17–36.

Torres, S. (1999) A culturally-relevant theoretical framework for the study of successful ageing, *Ageing and Society,* 19: 33–51.

Torres, S. (2001) *Understanding 'successful aging'*. Uppsala: Uppsala University, Department of Sociology.

Townsend, P. (1959) *The Family Life of Old People*. Harmondsworth: Penguin Books.

Townsend, P. (1979) *Poverty in the United Kingdom*. Harmondsworth: Penguin Books.

Townsend, P. and Walker, A. (1995) *The Future of Pensions: Revitalising National Insurance*. London: Fabian Society.

Trinder, C. (1990) *Employment after 55*, National Institute for Economic and Social Research discussion paper no. 166.

Tronti, L. (1998) Per il riordino degli ammortizzatori sociali, *Politica economica*, 1: 187–213.

Trossholmen, N. (2000) *Tid till eftertanke*. Skrifter från Etnologiska föreningen i Västsverige 32. Göteborg: Etnologiska Föreningen i Västsverige.

Trost, J. (1993) *Familjen i Sverige*. Stockholm: Liber Utbildning.

Trydegård, G-B. (1998) Public long term care in Sweden, *Journal of Gerontological Social Work*, 29(4): 13–34.

Trydegård, G-B. (2000) *Tradition, Change and Variation*. Stockholm: Stockholm University, Department of Social Work.

Trydegård, G-B. and Thorslund, M. (2001) Inequality in the welfare state? *International Journal of Social Welfare*, 10: 174–84.

Trydegård, G-B. and Thorslund, M. (2002) Explaining local variation in home-help services: The impact of path dependency in Swedish municipalities 1976–1997, in G-B Trydegård *Tradition, Change and Variation. Past and Present Trends in Public Old Age Care*. Diss. Stockholm: Department for Social Work, Stockholm University.

The Stationery Office (2002) *Social Trends*, Department of Health. London: The Stationery Office

The Stationery Office(2004) *Social Trends,* Department of Health, London: The Stationery Office.

Tune, R. and Bowie, P. (2000) The quality of residential and nursing-home care for people with dementia', *Age and Ageing*, 29: 325–28.

Tunstall, J. (1957) *Old and Alone*. London: Routledge & Kegan Paul.

Turrini, O. (1987) *Le Università della terza età. ISFOL*. Rome: Edizioni Lavoro.

Ueltzhöffer, J. (1999) *Generationenkonflikt und Generationenbündnis in der Bürgergesellschaft*. Stuttgart: Ministerium für Arbeit, Gesundheit und Sozialordnung.

Urbani, G. (1991) Introduzione, in *L'anziano attivo*. Torino: Giovanni Agnelli.

Veenhoven, R. (2000) The four qualities of life. Ordering concepts and measures of the good life, *Journal of Happiness Studies*, 1: 1–39.

Veer, A. de and Kerkstra, A. (1998) *Bewonerspanel verpleeghuizen*, Utrecht: NIVEL.

Verbrugge, L.M. (1995) New thinking and science on disability in mid- and late life, *European Journal of Public Health* 1: 20–8.

Victor, C., Bowling, A., Bond, J. and Scambler, S. (2003) *Loneliness, Social Isolation and Living Alone in Later Life*. Sheffield: Growing Older Programme, University of Sheffield.

Victor, C., Scambler, S., Bond, J., Bowling, A. (2000) Being alone in later life: loneliness, social isolation and living alone, *Reviews in Clinical Gerontology*, 10: 407–17.

Vitali, O. (2002) Rapporto 2001 sulla qualità della vita in Italia, *Italia Oggi*, *Documenti*, 15 January.

Vitali, O. (2003) Rapporto 2003 sulla qualità della vita in Italia, *Italia Oggi*, *Documenti*, December.

Wagner, M., Schütze, Y. and Lang, F.R. (1996) Soziale Beziehungen alter Menschen, in K.U. Mayer and P.B. Baltes (eds) *Die Berliner Altersstudie*. Berlin: Akademie-Verlag.

Wahl, H.-W. (1991) *'Das kann ich allein!' Selbständigkeit im Alter: Chancen und Grenzen*. Bern: Huber.

Wahl, H.-W., Mollenkopf, H. and Oswald, F. (1999) *Alte Menschen in ihrer Umwelt*. Wiesbaden: Westdeutscher Verlag.

Wahl, H.-W. and Reichert, M. (1991) Psychologische Forschung in Alten- und Altenpflegeheimen in den achtziger Jahren, *Zeitschrift für Gerontopsychologie und -psychiatrie*, 4: 233–55.

Walker, A. (1980) The social creation of poverty and dependency in old age, *Journal of Social Policy*, 9(1): 45–75.

Walker, A. (1981) Towards a political economy of old age, *Ageing and Society*, 1(1): 73–94.

Walker, A. (1982a) (ed.) *Community Care*. Oxford, Blackwell.

Walker, A. (1982b) Dependency and old age, *Social Policy and Administration*, 16(2): 116–37.

Walker, A. (1985) Early retirement: release or refuge from the labour market, *The Quarterly Journal of Social Affairs*, 1(3): 211–29.

Walker, A. (1993) *Age and Attitudes*. Brussels: European Commission.

Walker, A. (1997) *Combating Age Barriers in Employment*. Luxembourg: Office for Official Publications of the European Communities.

Walker, A. (1999) Public policy and theories of ageing: constructing and reconstructing old age, in V. Bengston and K. Schaie (eds) *Handbook of Theories of Ageing*. New York: Springer.

Walker, A. (1999) The future of pensions and retirement in Europe, *Hallym International Journal of Aging*, 1(2): 3–15.

Walker, A. (2002) A strategy for active ageing, *International Social Security Review*, 55(1): 121–39.

Walker, A. (2005) (ed.) *Understanding Quality of Life in Old Age*. Maidenhead: Open University Press.

Walker, A., Guillemard, A-M. and Alber, J. (1993) *Older People in Europe – Social and Economic Policies*. Brussels: European Commission.

Walker, A. and Hagan Hennessy, C. (2004) (eds.) *Growing Older: Quality of Life in Old Age*. Maidenhead: Open University Press.

Walker, A. and Maltby, T. (1997) *Ageing Europe*. Buckingham: Open University Press.

Walker, A. and Warren, L. (1996) *Changing Services for Older People*. Maidenhead: Open University Press.

Walter, H. (1999) *Vivere la vecchiaia. Sfide e nuove qualità di vita*. Rome: Edizioni Armando.

Walter, U. and Schwartz, F.W. (2001) Gesundheit der Älteren und Potenziale der Prävention und Gesundheitsförderung, in Deutsches Zentrum für Altersfragen (DZA) (ed.) *Personale, gesundheitliche und Umweltressourcen im Alter*, Band 1. Opladen: Leske & Budrich.

Weber G., Glück J., Sassenrath S. *et al.* (2003) *Self Resources in Advanced and Old Age*. Report to European Commission, Centre for Social Policy Research and Development, University of Wales, Bangor.

Weisser, G. (1972) Grundsätze der Verteilungspolitik, in B. Külp and W. Schreiber (eds), *Soziale Sicherheit.* Cologne, Berlin: Kiepenheuer & Witsch.

Wenger, C. and Burholt, V. (2001) Differences over time in older people's relationships with children, grandchildren, nieces and nephews in rural North Wales, *Ageing and Society*, 21: 567–90.

Wenger, C.G. (2001) Myths and realities of ageing in rural Britain, *Ageing and Society*, 21: 117–30.

Wenger, G.C. (1984) *The Supportive Network: Coping with Old Age*, London: Allen & Unwin.

Westergaard, J., Noble, I. and Walker, A. (1989) *After Redundancy*, Oxford: Polity Press.

Westerhof, G., Dittmann-Kohli, F. and Thissen, T. (2001) Beyond Life-Satisfaction, *Social Indicators Research*, 56: 179–203.

Westerhof, G.J. (2001a) Wohlbefinden in der zweiten Lebenshälfte, in F. Dittmann-Kohli, Ch. Bode and G.J. Westerhof (eds) *Die zweite Lebenshälfte*, Schriftenreihe des BFSFJ Band 195. Stuttgart: Kohlhammer.

Westerhof, G.J. (2001b) Arbeit und Beruf im persönlichen Sinnsystem, in F. Dittmann-Kohli, Ch. Bode and G.J. Westerhof (eds) *Die zweite Lebenshälfte*. Schriftenreihe des BFSFJ Band 195. Stuttgart: Kohlhammer.

Wever, I. (2000) *Het verzorgingshuis in twee varianten.* Utrecht: Nederlands instituut voor zorg en welzijn.

Wilkinson, R. (1999) *Unhealthy Societies.* London: Routledge.

Wilson, J.G., Calsyn, R.J. and Orlofsky, J.L. (1994) Impact of sibling relationships on social support and morale in the elderly, *Journal of Gerontological Social Work*, 22(3–4): 157–70.

Winqvist, M. (1999) *Vuxna barn med hjälpbehövande föräldrar – en livsforms-analys.* Uppsala: Uppsala universitet, Sociologiska institutionen.

Zank, S. and Baltes, M.M. (1994) Psychologische Interventionsmöglichkeiten in Altenheimen, in A. Kruse and H.-W. Wahl (eds) *Altern und Wohnen im Heim: Endstation oder Lebensort?* Bern: Huber.

Zank, S. and Baltes, M.M. (1998) Förderung von Selbständigkeit und Lebenszufriedenheit alter Menschen in stationären Einrichtungen, in A. Kruse (ed.) *Psychosoziale Gerontologie*, Band 2: Intervention. Göttingen: Hogrefe.

287

Zapf, D. (1991) Arbeit und Wohlbefinden, in A. Abele and P. Becker (eds) *Wohlbefinden: Theorie, Empirie, Diagnostik*. Weinheim: Juventa.

Zapf, W. (1984) Individuelle Wohlfahrt, in W. Glatzer and W. Zapf (eds) *Lebensqualität in der Bundesrepublik*. Frankfurt am Main: Campus.

Zapf, W. (ed.) (1994) Technik, Alter, Lebensqualität. Schriftenreihe des Bundesministeriums für Familie und Senioren, Band 23. Stuttgart: Kohlhammer.

Zapf, W., Schupp, J. and Habich, R. (eds) (1996) *Lebenslagen im Wandel*. Frankfurt am Main, New York: Campus.

Zimmer, Z. and Chappell, N. (1999) Receptivity to new technology among older adults, *Disability and Rehabilitation*, 21(5/6): 222–30.

Zuliani, A. (2000) *Salute e Sistema Sanitario in Italia negli anni '90*. Paper presented at the University of Bologna on 1 December. www.istat.it/novita/farmzul.pdf.

Index

Page numbers in *italics* refer to tables; *n* indicates a chapter note; *passim* refers to numerous scattered mentions within page range.

AGEING IN THE CITY
Everyday Life in Poor Neighbourhoods

Thomas Scharf, Chris Phillipson and Allison E. Smith

This book addresses key issues associated with the experience of ageing in Britain's deprived urban neighbourhoods, examining factors such as poverty, crime, social problems, community and local services. It draws upon original empirical research including detailed interviews with 130 older people living in deprived neighbourhoods. This rich data is supplemented where appropriate with findings drawn from a survey of an additional 600 older people in the same communities.

The book discusses what it means to be growing older in the city, and how poverty and neighbourhood issues impact on individuals. Importantly, it also discusses future recommendations for social policy in this important area.

Ageing in the City is key reading for undergraduate and postgraduate courses in social gerontology, urban studies, social geography, social anthropology, community care, social policy and sociology.

Contents:
Introduction: setting the scene – Ageing in urban environments - Everyday lives of older people - Perceptions of the neighbourhood - Poverty and deprivation - Social relationships - Using services - Quality of life in urban areas - Conclusion and policy implications - Index.

c.192pp   0 335 21515 7 (Paperback)   0 335 21516 5 (Hardback)

GROWING OLDER
Quality of Life in Old Age

Alan Walker and Catherine Hagan Hennessy

This volume introduces the work of the Economic and Social Research Council (ESRC) funded Growing Older Programme (1999-2004) and provides a showcase for the other volumes in the series. It focuses on ways in which quality of life can be extended for older people and offers short research-based summaries of key findings on a variety of core topics with a major emphasis on the views of older people themselves..

Many of the leading names in social gerontology in the United Kingdom have contributed their findings, providing the most up-to-date and broad-ranging information available on quality of life in old age. Topics discussed include:

- Defining and measuring quality of life

- Inequalities in quality of life

- Technology and the built environment

- Healthy and active ageing

- Family and support networks

- Participation and grandparenthood

Growing Older is suitable for undergraduate and postgraduate students of social gerontology, sociology and social policy. It is of interest to professionals working with older people, including social workers, gerontology nurses and community support workers. There are also important findings for policy-makers.

Contributors:
Sara Arber; Madhavi Bajekal; David Blane; John Bond; Ann Bowling; Jabeer Butt; Lynda Clarke; Joanne Cook; Kate Davidson; Murna Downs; Zahava Gabriel; Ini Grewal; Catherine Hagan Hennessey; Caroline Holland; Gill Hubbard; Leonie Kellaher; Charlotte MacDonald; Tony Maltby; Jo Moriarty; Joan Murphy; James Nazroo; Sheila M. Peace; Chris Phillipson; Ceridwen Roberts; Sasha Scambler; Thomas Scharf; Allison Smith; Susan Tester; Christina Victor; Alan Walker; Lorna Warren.

Contents:
Contributors - Preface - Introducing the Growing Older Programme on extending quality of life - Quality of life in old age from the perspectives of older people - Ethnic inequalities - Environment, identity and old age: Quality of life or a life of quality? - Poverty and social exclusion: Growing older in deprived urban neighbourhoods - Loneliness in later life - Older men: Their health behaviours and partnership status - A participatory approach to older women's quality of life - Social support and ethnicity in old age - The meaning of grandparenthood, and its contribution to the quality of life of older people - Frailty and institutional life - Conclusion - Bibliography - Index.

c.280pp   0 335 21507 6 (Paperback)   0 335 21508 4 (Hardback)

UNDERSTANDING QUALITY OF LIFE IN OLD AGE

Alan Walker (ed)

This book considers key findings from the Economic and Social Research Council (ESRC) funded Growing Older Programme (1999-2004) and presents these in a lively thematic format. It discusses topics such as environment, family, bereavement, identity, and social interaction and describes key concepts and measures. Using data drawn from a range of different research projects, the chapters illustrate considerable methodological diversity to capture a broad picture of quality of life for older people. Key implications for future research on quality of life in older age are also proposed.

The book is a companion volume to *Growing Older: Quality of Life in Old Age* edited by Alan Walker and Catherine Hagan Hennessy and is recommended reading on a range of advanced under-graduate and postgraduate courses including social gerontology, social work, sociology and social policy.

Contributors:
Sara Arber, John Baldock, Kate M. Bennett, David Blane, Ann Bowling, Elizabeth Breeze, Jabeer Butt, Lynda Clarke, Peter Coleman, Kate Davidson, Murna Downs, Maria Evandrou, Ken Gilhooly, Mary Gilhooly, Jane Gow, Jan Hadlow, Catherine Hagan Hennessy, Paul Higgs, Caroline Holland, Georgina M. Hughes, Martin Hyde, Leonie Kellaher, Mary Maynard, Kevin McKee, F. McKiernan, Christopher McKevitt, Marie Mills, Jo Moriarty, James Nazroo, Sheila Peace, Thomas Scharf, Philip T. Smith, Peter Speck, Susan Tester, Christina Victor, Alan Walker, Peter Warr, Lorna Warren, Dick Wiggins, Fiona Wilson.

Contents:
Investigating quality of life in the Growing Older Programme - Quality of life: meaning and measure-ment - Dimensions of the inequalities in quality of life in older age - Getting out and about - Family and economic roles - Social involvement: aspects of gender and ethnicity - Social isolation and loneli-ness - Frailty, identity and the quality of later life - Identity, meaning and social support - Elderly bereaved spouses: issues of belief, well-being and support - Conclusion: from research to action - Index.

c.192pp   0 335 21523 8 (Paperback)   0 335 21524 6 (Hardback)

SEXUALITY, SEXUAL HEALTH AND AGEING

Merryn Gott

- What factors underpin dominant understandings of later life sexuality?

- How do older people experience and prioritise sexuality and sexual health?

- What sexual health issues are relevant to older people and how are these addressed by health care professionals?

This is the first book to integrate theoretical insights into sexuality, sexual health and ageing, with research findings from studies conducted with older people and the professionals that work with them.

The book is split into three sections. In the first section stereotypes that typify contemporary understandings of sexuality and ageing are explored, particularly the 'myth of asexual old age' and the more recent stereotype of the 'sexy oldie'. Section two identifies what we actually know about ageing and sexuality by reviewing current literature, as well as presenting findings from one of the first qualitative studies to explore sexuality from the perspective of older people themselves. The final section of the book explores what 'sexual health' means within the context of ageing and focuses on issues relevant to health professionals working with older people.

Sexuality, Sexual Health and Ageing provides key reading for students, researchers, practitioners and policymakers working within gerontology, sociology, psychology, social work, health sciences, nursing and medicine. This book is likely to become essential reading for all academics and professionals working with older people or in the area of sexual health.

Contents:
*Introduction – **Section 1: Exploring understandings of sexuality and ageing** – Why are sexuality and old age incompatible? Unpicking the myth of the 'asexual old age' – The 'sexy oldie': The creation of new myths about sexuality and ageing – **Section 2: Focusing upon older people's experiences of sexuality and ageing** – What do we 'know' about sexuality and ageing? – How important is sex to older people? – Diversity and later life sexuality – **Section 3: Sexual health, sexual problems and ageing** – Sexual risk-taking and sexually transmitted infections in later life – Sexual 'dysfunctions' and ageing – Health professional attitudes towards later life sexuality and sexual health – Index.*

c.208pp   0 335 21018 X (Paperback)   0 335 21019 8 (Hardback)